Books can h

"Books on Pr

Smoking is the si... 'k perio

which remains the UK's big...

your risk of developing heart disease drama... renewed

quit smoking for good. The British Heart Foundation

welcomes this book, which we are sure will provide excen

for smokers trying to give up and will help protect many people's long-

term heart health.'

Dr Mike Knapton, Director of Prevention and Care, British Heart
Foundation

'With clearly presented facts and a whole host of useful tips and hints,
this indispensable book will guide the reader step by step through the
whole process of stopping smoking. The information about smoking
and quitting is clearly presented, making this a really useful tool for
anyone who wants to give up for good.'

Christine Owens, Head of Tobacco Control, The Roy Castle Lung
Cancer Foundation

'Planning your quit attempt can be the key to success. *You Can Stop
Smoking* will give you all the tools you need to free yourself from
addiction for good. The methods have been tried and trusted by
the hundreds of thousands of smokers who have used the support
of the NHS, and Jennifer Percival helps you to use these methods
successfully. No Smoking Day would recommend this book to anyone
who wants to turn their back on cigarettes for good. You *can* stop
smoking and this book gives you everything you need to be a success.'

Ben Youdan, Chief Executive, No Smoking Day

'This book needs to be read by every person who smokes, and I really
hope that it will result in a huge leap in the number of people who
successfully manage to give up the habit – for good. Jennifer Percival
has worked for the Royal College of Nursing for a number of years,
at local, national and international levels. She is highly respected by
her colleagues, and we believe that Jennifer has made an outstanding
contribution to society by supporting smokers to quit.'

Lynn Young, Primary Care Advisor, Royal College of Nursing

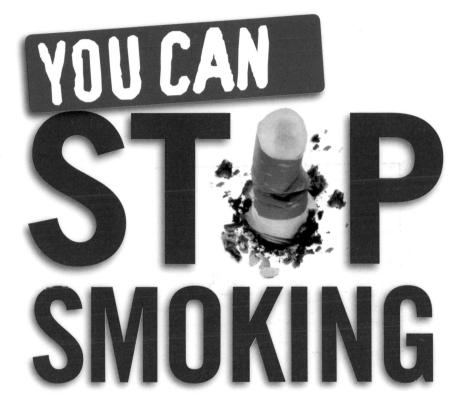

YOU CAN STOP SMOKING

Jennifer Percival

In association with
NHS Innovations London

First published in Great Britain in 2007 by
Virgin Books Ltd
Thames Wharf Studios
Rainville Road
London
W6 9HA

A catalogue record for this book is available from the British
Library.

ISBN 978 0 75351 143 5

The paper used in this book is a natural, recyclable
product made from wood grown in sustainable forests. The
manufacturing process conforms to the regulations of the
country of origin.

Designed & typeset by Virgin Books Ltd

Printed and bound in Great Britain

Contents

This book is dedicated to my son, Alexander, in the hope he and every other teenager in the world chooses a smoke-free life.

Acknowledgements

I would like to thank everyone who supported the production of You Can Stop Smoking, especially Dr Dawn Milner who provided valuable advice and moral support throughout the process of researching, writing and editing the material.

Special thanks also go to the dedicated staff of the NHS Stop Smoking Services who took the time to share their tips and smokers' stories with me.

I would like to acknowledge Isobel Abbott, Caroline Douglas, Flis McDonald, Dawn Levin, Kerry Lynch, Alison Nichol, Mohammed Patel, Alexia Paterson, Jenny Pool, Dawn Powers, Janet Pratt, Robert Smith, Gay Sutherland and Jo Woodvine for their kind help.

Finally, this project was brought together by the dedicated team at NHS Innovations London and a special mention goes to Adam Daykin.

About the author

Jennifer Percival currently runs the Royal College of Nursing's Tobacco Education Project and is the specialist nurse for the Department of Health's TV Testimonial campaign. Jennifer is a qualified nurse, midwife and health visitor who holds diplomas in counseling and teaching. She worked for over 20 years in the NHS, before specialising in health promotion and public health. She was awarded a Winston Churchill Fellowship in 1990 and visited Australia to study their methods of helping people stop smoking.

Foreword
Richard Branson

Giving up smoking is one of the best things I've ever done. You may not believe it, but it's one of my proudest achievements. By buying this book you've taken the first step towards one of the most positive, life-changing decisions you'll ever make.

I'm not going to pretend it's easy to quit the cigarettes, and all of us need a helping hand sometimes. And that's what's so great about this book – it's a personal companion to guide you through the process of giving up for good.

The key to giving up successfully, like in so many areas of life, is preparation. Set a quit date in advance and you'll have something to work towards. Know how you're going to deal with the cravings and you'll be able to get through even the most stressful situations without automatically reaching for the fags.

This book is full of straightforward but inspirational advice to help you quit for life, and most importantly lets you tailor a programme that's right for you. But don't try and go it alone – get your friends and family on board and tell them why it's so important that they support you. And whatever you do, don't let anyone put you off (or turn you on!).

Finally, be proud of your success and celebrate every target you reach. Every goal, no matter how small it may seem, deserves a reward. So, whether it's one week or six months without a cigarette, treat yourself.

Good luck.

Richard Branson

Introduction

⟩ How can this book help?

This book contains everything you need to know in order to successfully give up smoking for life. By reading this book and following the step-by-step plan, you can look forward to a healthier, happier – and slightly richer! – future as a non-smoker.

But it won't all be plain sailing. If you or someone you know has ever tried to quit smoking you'll know how tough it can be. The cycle of addiction can be difficult to break and many people will try five or six times to quit before they succeed.

The good news is that with a little careful planning and the right information and support, giving up can be far more simple and painless than you thought. And that's where this book can really help.

You Can Stop Smoking will arm you with all the knowledge you need to successfully ditch the cigarettes for good. It'll be your companion on your journey from smoker to non-smoker. It won't lecture or talk down to you or try and scare you with shocking statistics or baffle you with medical jargon.

Rather, it will give you the confidence to successfully quit smoking and help you look forward to a smoke-free future. Most importantly, everything in this book is based on tried and tested methods which have helped thousands of people to give up.

But every journey begins with a first step, and in this case that first step is the decision to stop smoking. It's up to you to make that decision, and only you can say if you're ready to give up. But if you're reading this and pondering whether the time is right for you, I would encourage you to go ahead and make that decision.

And with a total ban on smoking in workplaces, including bars and clubs, coming into force in the UK by July 2007, there's never been a better time to quit. In fact, according to a

No Smoking Day survey, over 2.8 million of the UK's smokers say they'll give up as a result of the ban. So if you do want to quit you're in good company!

In this book you'll find out how to:

- **set your 'quit date' and plan your personal campaign to quit**
- **deal with nicotine withdrawal and cravings**
- **manage those difficult first few days of not smoking**
- **enlist the help of others**
- **live a healthy, smoke-free life!**

Why delay?

Everyone knows smoking can cause potentially fatal illnesses – it says so on the packet in big, black letters! But ask any smoker why they don't want to quit and you'll hear the same excuses over and over again: smoking relaxes me and helps me concentrate; I only smoke five a day; my granddad smoked all his life and never got ill; I could be hit by a bus tomorrow; I'm young and healthy, I'll think about giving up later.

But what if all the 'good' things about smoking weren't true or were based on falsehood and myths? What if smoking didn't relax you at all, but in fact had the opposite effect? What if smoking actually had no effect at all on your concentration? What if just a single cigarette a day tripled your risk of lung cancer?

The truth is there are no 'good' things about smoking, and the negative effects far outweigh any possible positives. Sure, we all know someone who smoked until they were 80 years old and never got ill. But the fact is that over 100,000 people in the UK die every year as a direct result of smoking. That's 13 people every hour. And smoking is by far the greatest single cause of preventable disease and premature death in the UK.

Many long-term smokers say that cigarettes are like an old friend, and that giving up will be like losing that friendship. Even the phrase 'giving up' suggests loss. But it's important not to think like this. After all, you haven't always been a smoker, have you? You're simply going back to how you were before you started smoking. And you'll be a lot better off for it – both in terms of your health and your bank balance!

❯ How does this book work?

You Can Stop Smoking is split into clear and easy to follow chapters which form a step-by-step plan to guide you through the process of giving up. You'll find a number of questionnaires and interactive elements in the book which will help you personalise your plan to quit.

Part one is all about preparing to quit – from setting the all important 'quit date' and enlisting help and support from other people – and contains all the information you need on nicotine replacement therapy and other treatments available to you.

Part two guides you through the crucial first few days and weeks of being a non-smoker and contains all the information you'll need to maintain your new smoke-free life.

So turn the page and begin a new chapter in your life. By the time you finish reading this book I hope you'll be able to say with confidence 'I'm a non-smoker (and I plan to stay that way)!'

An ex-smoker's story

'I always thought if I had a good enough reason to stop smoking then I would. Like many smokers I used to think, "I could get knocked down by a bus." The "bus" hit me on 23 November 2004 when I had a heart attack. Believe me, when you are in that situation you wish you were a non-smoker. It's hard to believe now but that morning, with a dull ache in my chest, I still "lit up" in the car! We all think we are invincible and "it won't happen to me". Well, unfortunately, it does. My husband and daughters have been wonderful. At the time my 15-year-old had tried smoking, as many kids of her age do, and I'm sure that she would have become a smoker had we not had to go through this as a family. I'm so pleased now my life is not ruled by my next cigarette. Going out is a pleasure because I'm not thinking about the next cigarette and

where to have it. You can't imagine how horrible you smell until you stop smoking, it's really awful. I love non-smoking venues now! I am much less stressed – smoking adds to stress and certainly does not help it. I walk miles, go to exercise class and am even thinking of taking up cycling. I can run now and not be gasping to breathe. I'm really glad I don't smoke any more. I've gained a little weight but perhaps the cycling might get rid of that! I now say to every smoker I meet, "Stopping smoking can have a positive effect on your life – give it a try!"' Jackie Groves

Part 1
PLANNING
TO
QUIT

'You are about to
set off on a new
journey...'

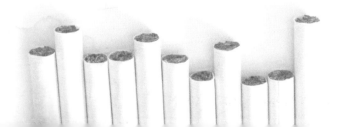

Chapter 1
Sign Up To Our Plan
– And Stop Smoking For Good!

So, you've read the introduction, decided that you'd like to give up and are wondering what to do next. Don't panic. This book is here to help. *You Can Stop Smoking* is based on well-proven techniques that have helped thousands of smokers stop smoking – and stay stopped. They benefited, and you can too.

But just in case there are any little doubts about giving up still lingering in the back of your mind this chapter will explain the enormous benefits of quitting, and the harmful effects of carrying on. It will encourage you to examine your reasons for smoking, and debunk some myths about the 'advantages' of cigarettes. You'll also learn a few facts about your habit. But don't worry, there are no lectures. You know when the time is right – and it's not when you're put under pressure.

I'm not going to pretend that giving up smoking is easy, but it can be done. *You Can Stop Smoking* will make the task as painless and effective as possible. To reinforce your resolve let's start by explaining why giving up is such a good idea.

An ex-smoker's story

'I was coughing up some really bad gunk, my fingers were numb, and I felt tired and unwell all the time. I thought it's time I stopped smoking. The advert on TV – where fat drops out of a cigarette – really hit home. I thought, "That's my arteries and I've got to stop smoking."' Andy Cook

---

❯ Health benefits of giving up smoking

The great news is that, from the very moment you stub out your last cigarette, your body begins an amazing journey of recovery. Here's what happens:

20 minutes   Blood pressure and pulse return to normal.

Circulation improves, especially in hands and feet.

8 hours   Blood oxygen levels increase to normal.

Your chances of having a heart attack start to fall.

24 hours   Carbon monoxide leaves the body.

The lungs start to clear out mucus and debris.

48 hours   Your body is now nicotine-free.

Your senses of taste and smell begin to improve.

72 hours   Breathing is easier, and your energy levels increase.

2–12 weeks   Circulation improves throughout your body.

Walking and exercise get easier.

3–9 months   Breathing problems, coughing, shortness of breath and wheezing improve.

Lung efficiency increases by 5–10 per cent.

Reduced disease risk

Giving up smoking reduces the risk of developing a host of smoking-related illnesses. If you give up at the age of 30 you'll gain an average of 10 more years of life. After 15 years of giving up, your risk of developing lung cancer is only slightly greater than someone who has never smoked. It's good news, too, for people with heart disease. When smokers give up, their symptoms of heart disease improve and the risk of heart attack is reduced. For those who have had a heart attack, stopping smoking will reduce the risk of a second one.

Giving up smoking also hastens your recovery from illness, reduces the risk of further complications and extends life expectancy. Lung function improves and your capacity for exercise increases. Stopping smoking at any age extends life expectancy, provided you stop before you develop cancer or other serious disease. Even if damage has been done, you'll still benefit from stopping. Here is the day-to-day cost of smoking:

Boosting lung function

Lung function – the ability of the lungs to do their job – is affected by the number of cigarettes you smoke and how long you have been smoking. The good news is that the rate at which older ex-smokers are diagnosed with respiratory symptoms, such as coughing, wheezing and excess phlegm, declines from the moment they stop smoking.

Although some types of lung damage after years of smoking may be permanent, stopping definitely prevents the damage getting worse. For some smokers, this makes the difference between living an independent life and spending the rest of your years housebound and on a permanent oxygen supply.

❯ Disadvantages of smoking

Physical Problems
- Wheezing, shortness of breath, cough.
- Lack of energy, poor concentration.
- Reduced fertility and more risky pregnancy.
- Bad breath, common in heavy smokers.
- Gum disease, tooth decay, tooth loss and ulcers.
- Damaged taste buds and stained teeth.

Social Issues
- Increased risk of fire in the home.
- Harm to others in the family, including family pets.
- Stained walls and tobacco smoke make your home harder to sell.

Financial
- High cost – over £2,000 per year for a 20-a-day smoker.
- Less money for unexpected bills.

Emotional
- Being a sexual turn-off to people who do not smoke.
- Feeling constantly controlled by cigarettes.
- Ever-present nagging sense of guilt/health worries.
- Increasing pressure from a smoke-free society.

Vanity
- Hair, hands and clothes smelling of smoke.
- Skin damaged by smoke – greyish, wasted appearance.
- Puckering lines around the mouth from drawing on cigarettes.
- Premature skin ageing – you look 10 to 20 years older.

⊘ The effect of smoking on lung function

This graph shows how a smoker's lungs work less effectively than a non-smoker's.

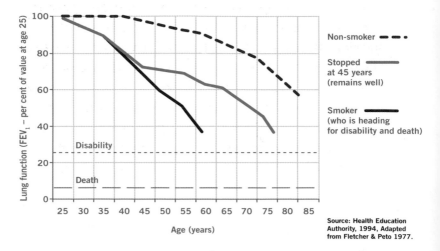

Source: Health Education Authority, 1994, Adapted from Fletcher & Peto 1977.

⊘ The effects on children

Second-hand tobacco smoke affects others too – especially children. The young are vulnerable because their bodies are still developing. Their bronchial tubes and lungs are smaller and immune systems less developed, so they are more prone to infection. They breathe faster than adults, taking in proportionally more chemicals than an adult per kilogram of body weight. Smoking near children causes asthma attacks and increases the risk of wheezing, coughing, phlegm and breathlessness. Second-hand smoke is a cause of bronchitis and pneumonia in children and increases their risk of meningitis.

In households where both parents smoke, young children have a 72 per cent increased risk of respiratory illnesses. Parental smoking causes acute and chronic middle ear disease in children – often leading to deafness. Babies and children exposed to a smoky atmosphere are more likely to need hospital care in the first year of life and are also off sick from school more often due to coughs, colds and wheezing. Cot death is twice as likely in babies whose mothers smoke.

⊙ Preventing chronic lung disease

One of the worst smoking-related conditions is chronic obstructive pulmonary (lung) disease (COPD), which includes chronic bronchitis and emphysema. This progressively disabling disease is very rare in non-smokers. COPD can cause a great deal of suffering. Because of smoking, the small airways get narrowed or blocked and many of the tiny air sacs in the lung are destroyed. This makes it increasingly difficult to breathe properly. The onset of the disease is very gradual and breathlessness only becomes troublesome when about half of the lung is destroyed. Once the disease becomes established it is very difficult to reverse the problem – so the answer is to stop smoking before it starts.

An ex-smoker's story

Janice appears in a TV campaign to encourage smokers to quit. She is a very attractive lady who needs piped oxygen 24 hours a day. She looks at the camera and says, 'My name's Janice and the reason I've got these tubes is for oxygen to breathe.' Janice suffers from chronic obstructive pulmonary disease caused by her smoking. She is divorced and has three children. All her children take part in a care rota, taking turns to look after her, as she no longer has enough 'puff' even to comb her hair. Janice started smoking at an early age – 12 years old. She made several unsuccessful attempts before finally giving up for good at the age of 38. Her specialist had told her that if she didn't quit, she wouldn't survive to see her children grow up.

'I started because everybody was smoking. When I finally quit, I was annoyed at how easy I found it to stop. I wish I'd quit a hell of a lot sooner. I am a strong person; I can't believe I let something as small as a cigarette beat me.'

Because of her diseased lungs, Janice has had to have two major lung-reduction operations. Now she cannot talk or walk without oxygen. She is unable to get dressed, wash her hair, bathe or get into bed without help. She can't cook, climb stairs or undertake any physical activity. No one with even a slight cold can come near her and she is housebound during autumn and winter. Her breathing is affected by strong smells such as perfume and new paint. She can never go into a smoky environment, such as a pub or restaurant, or let anyone smoke in her home. At really bad times, she can't walk ten steps – even with oxygen.

'I can't go outside as the cold and damp air literally take my breath away. I hate winter – summer is really the only time for me.'

Janice is fully aware of the impact on her family. Her eldest daughter gave up her career to care for her full-time. She's also aware of all she misses out on because of her illness – her job, the opportunity to meet a new partner and just being able to pick up her granddaughter.

'They say life begins at 40 – but mine just went into a downhill spiral. Cigarettes are awful things. They take over your mind and your life.' Despite the burden of her disease, Janice manages to keep a positive outlook, saying, *'My situation's never going to change or get better but my children keep me going. They are my rock.'* Janice Matthews

⊘ What's in a cigarette?

You might think that cigarettes are nothing more than little paper tubes filled with chopped up tobacco with a filter at one end. The truth is that cigarettes contain a whole host of chemicals and substances that can be damaging to your health.

Tobacco leaf

Cigarettes contain cured tobacco leaf and the plant stem as well as 'fillers', which are made from the stems and other bits of tobacco which would otherwise be waste products. These are mixed with water and various flavourings and additives.

Additives

The tobacco industry puts additives into many of their products. These include humectants (moisturisers) which prolong shelf life; sugars which make the smoke seem milder and easier to inhale; salts to make the tobacco burn evenly; and flavourings such as chocolate and vanilla. While these sound quite harmless, in fact they may be toxic in combination with other substances. The full list of 600 permitted additives can be viewed on the Department of Health's website.

Chemicals

There are many gases, chemicals and metals in tobacco and tobacco smoke which are harmful to your health. These include

- **Acetone – found in nail polish remover**
- **Ammonia – used in tear gas and strong cleaning fluids**
- **Arsenic – a deadly poison used in insecticides**
- **Benzene – can cause cancer and is used as an industrial solvent**
- **Cadmium – a highly poisonous metal used in batteries**
- **Ethanol – used in anti-freeze**
- **Formaldehyde – used as an embalming fluid**
- **Hydrogen cyanide – one of the most toxic chemicals in cigarette smoke. It can cause headaches, nausea, dizziness and vomiting**
- **Nitrosamines – can cause cancer in humans and animals.**

Tar

Tar is the sticky brown substance that stains smokers' fingers and teeth yellowy brown and is made up of hundreds of different chemicals. When a smoker inhales, about 70 per cent of the tar contained in the smoke stays in their lungs. Many of the substances in tar are known to cause cancer and to damage the lungs and the small hairs (cilia) which help protect the lungs from dirt and infection.

Carbon monoxide (CO)

Carbon monoxide is a poisonous, odourless and tasteless gas which in large amounts is rapidly fatal. It is also found in high concentrations in cigarette smoke, as well as in car exhaust fumes and in the fumes from faulty gas appliances.

When you inhale tobacco smoke, carbon monoxide takes the place of oxygen in the blood, and this stops the cells and tissues from getting the oxygen needed to work properly and lowers the oxygen in the bloodstream by up to 20 per cent.

CO cuts down the efficiency of a smoker's breathing and may also be linked to the development of coronary heart disease and other major circulation problems. It is especially harmful during pregnancy as it reduces the amount of oxygen carried to the womb and developing baby.

Nicotine

Most smokers become dependent on the nicotine in cigarettes. Nicotine is as addictive as drugs such as heroin and cocaine, and cigarettes are highly efficient nicotine delivery devices.

Nicotine produces many effects on the body, including increasing the heart rate, the blood pressure, stimulating the central nervous system and speeding up the metabolism. Nicotine also affects the mood and behaviour of the smoker in a complex way. But nicotine does not cause cancer.

Reducing or stopping nicotine intake can cause a number of withdrawal symptoms, including depressed mood, insomnia, irritability, frustration or anger, anxiety, difficulty with concentration, restlessness, decreased heart rate, dizziness and increased appetite.

Many smokers believe that a cigarette helps them to relax. The reality is that the nicotine 'hit' satisfies the body's craving. This is a classic cycle of addiction – craving followed by satisfaction followed by withdrawal. When this cycle is repeated many times a day it is easy to understand just how addictive smoking is and how difficult it is for smokers to quit.

❯ See how cigarettes affect your body

Try these practical exercises to check what is happening to your body each time you smoke a cigarette.

Feel your pulse

○ Just before you light up, check your pulse by placing your index finger firmly on the smooth area on the inside of your wrist. Count your pulse for a minute. A normal pulse beats 60–80 times a minute. What is your rate? Note this number   .

○ Immediately after you put out a cigarette, take your pulse again   . You'll find that your pulse rate has increased. This shows how smoking affects the heart.

See the tar

○ Inhale from a cigarette as normal and then put the cigarette down. Take a white tissue and hold it tightly over your mouth. Blow out the smoke you've taken into your lungs. See how much of a yellow mark it leaves on the tissue. (It may not be very much.)

○ Take in another mouthful of smoke and, without inhaling into your lungs, blow it out through a clean tissue. You'll see a circle of brown tar. Note the difference between the two tissues. You're looking at visible proof of how much tar stays in your lungs. If you smoke 20 cigarettes a day, week in, week out, you'll see why breathing problems occur.

How steady is your hand?

○ Try doing a delicate task just before and after smoking a cigarette. For example, try building a tower of children's bricks or threading a needle. After having a cigarette you may well find that your hand is trembling and it's hard to keep it steady.

⟩ Check your blood pressure

Measure your blood pressure before and after a cigarette. Most high street pharmacists and GP surgeries offer blood pressure monitoring for free. You may well find your blood pressure has become raised after smoking.

⟩ Measure your carbon monoxide

Carbon monoxide (CO) is a harmful gas produced by burning tobacco. It is breathed into the lungs by all smokers when they inhale tobacco smoke. CO gets readily absorbed into the bloodstream where it reduces the release of oxygen from the red blood cells. Smokers have up to 20 per cent of their normal blood oxygen replaced by CO. This means the heart has to work harder and smokers can get breathless when they exert themselves. CO also makes the blood thicker, which causes a fatty build up inside the arteries.

When you stop smoking, the level of CO in your blood falls almost immediately and can be the same as a non-smoker's within a few days. Why not ask for a CO reading from your doctor or other health care professional? It may help you decide to quit smoking. If you repeat the test regularly after you quit, you will see immediate proof that your efforts have been rewarded, which will strengthen your resolve to keep going.

An ex-smoker's story

'I was a chain smoker but have now kicked the filthy habit! I got the support I needed from fellow quitters. I am no longer sick and tired of feeling sick and tired. I can breathe without wheezing. I can sleep normally and I appreciate food more. I'm a born-again non-smoker. My motto now is "not one puff ever". My health has improved tremendously. It hasn't been easy and every day is a trial, but one has to take it a day at a time. Being part of a group of ex-smokers has been a great help. My energy levels have improved, I no longer cough in the morning, and my house and clothes smell great.' Jerry Martin

---

❯ How important is smoking to you?

There are advantages and disadvantages with almost every habit. People who decide to continue smoking often become fixated on the perceived 'advantages' and ignore the disadvantages. Before you can consider stopping you'll need to believe the benefits are worth it. The following exercise invites you to make a deeper analysis of why you might want to continue smoking and the benefits of stopping.

❯ Record your current thoughts and beliefs

	Staying a Smoker	Stopping Smoking
Advantages	It's part of my life	Less nagging from my kids
Disadvantages	Work going smoke free soon	My way of dealing with stress and difficult situations

Are you thinking about making a change?

Write your personal assessment or conclusion below

Are you ready to stop?

What I like about smoking	My reasons for stopping
1	
2	
3	
4	
5	
6	
7	
8	
9	
10	

Do you want to stop smoking? Circle one answer.

YES   NO   MAYBE

⟩ Can you make the decision stop?

Before you set a date to stop smoking, you need to feel motivated and confident about this decision. The following exercise will help you find out how far along you are in the decision-making process. It will also show you what might still get in your way and the barriers you have to overcome.

On a scale of 1 to 10, how important is it for you to stop smoking?

Circle the number you have chosen

(Low) 1   2   3   4   5   6   7   8   9   10   (High)

What has happened to make you choose this number and not a lower one?

What would have to change for you to move to a higher number?

On a scale of 1 to 10, how confident do you feel about stopping smoking?

Circle the number you have chosen

(Low) 1   2   3   4   5   6   7   8   9   10   (High)

What has happened to make you choose this number and not a lower one?

What would need to happen to increase or maintain your CONFIDENCE to stop smoking?

What do you think are the main reasons you smoke?
Circle all that apply.

Habit   Addiction   Pleasure   Comfort
Relaxation   Social   Other reason?

❯ Keep a smoking record before you stop

Do you know how many you light up when you don't have a
strong desire to do so? This exercise will help you understand
more about why you smoke when you do and which cigarettes
are important to you. Keep a record of each cigarette you smoke
over a few days and the reason why. Include a typical mix of
work and social times. Rate each smoke on a scale of 1 to 5 for
enjoyment/value.

Time	Reason for smoking	How important is this cigarette 1= Not Very 5= Essential

Time	Reason for smoking	How important is this cigarette 1= Not Very 5= Essential

Coping strategies

Now work out strategies to manage, without lighting up, the times numbered 4–5.

The cigarettes I worry about missing are:	What else I might do at those times
1	
2	
3	
4	
5	

Learning from past experiences

If you've tried to stop smoking before, you will have some idea of what to expect next time around. This exercise helps you remember what worked for you in the past so you can build on these positive experiences.

Times I've given up smoking before	How long I stayed stopped?
1	
2	
3	
4	
5	

Thinking over the times you stopped in the past, how did you do it? Which strategies were the most successful? List the answers below.

What helped me to stop	What things got in my way?
1	
2	
3	
4	
5	

How did you cope physically during the time that you were off tobacco?

How did you feel mentally?

Emotionally – how did you handle not smoking?

Is anything from the past concerning you about or likely to get in the way of your next quit attempt?

❯ Are you planning a smoke-free life?

Use this page to keep a note of your thoughts so far.

I started smoking when I was _____ years old.

I've now been smoking for _____ years.

Currently I smoke _____ cigarettes a day.

I have probably smoked over _____ cigarettes in my life.

I now spend _____ a week on tobacco.

My main reason for being a smoker is

_____

_____

_____

_____

I'd like to quit smoking because

_____

_____

_____

_____

I am thinking of stopping on _____ (Date)

When I have stopped, I hope to feel

_____

_____

_____

Planning to go smoke free

One thing I will no longer have to worry about is

The people who will be really pleased with me are

I will be proud of myself because

It will be worth the effort because

❯ Delaying the decision to quit?

So far this section has concentrated on helping you gather more information on your smoking habit to help you decide what you want to do about it. If you have any doubts or have decided to put your plans to stop smoking on hold, please ask yourself why.

Are you unsure that you can do it?

Be assured, thousands of people manage to stop smoking each year. Ex-smokers are usually willing to share their experiences and advice. Will it help you to speak to someone you know who has successfully given up? It may also help to discuss your concerns with an advisor from the NHS Smoking Helpline 0800 169 0 169.

Do you think you lack the willpower?

Stopping smoking requires you to change many aspects of your life. Willpower is only a small part of the process. Take a second look at the people you know who have stopped smoking. Is there something different about them that makes you think only someone like them can do it? No, I didn't think so. If they can do it – so can you. All you need is to be prepared to work at each of the challenges along the way.

Is it because someone close to you still smokes?

Discuss the consequences to your quit attempt if they still smoke around you when you stop. It is possible for others to support you even though they choose to remain smokers. All they need do to help is change some of their habits, such as not lighting up in front of you, smoking outside, and not offering you a cigarette.

Are you are waiting for a friend or family member to join you?

You have to stop smoking for yourself. Only you will know when the time is right. If you are ready and your partner is not, make time to explain your reasons why stopping now is important to you. Ask them if they will join you. If they say 'no', and you can't reach a compromise, you have the following options:

○ Choose a new date when they can agree to support you.

○ Go for your goal without their support.

Are you trying to accommodate another person? Circle one.

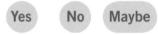

Before you abandon the idea of stopping smoking, ask yourself, 'Is this person important enough for me to risk continuing to smoke.' If 'yes', ask yourself if you may resent them for it later on and, if so, how that might affect your future relationship.

An ex-smoker's story

'I started smoking when I was 17. I'm now in my fifties and last year I had three strokes. I got so bad I couldn't walk down the road. My doctor said that if I had another stroke it would kill me and I had to stop smoking immediately. It hasn't been easy. I've had a horrible year and a personal tragedy to cope with but I've still not gone back to smoking. If I can do it, anyone can. I've just kept going one day at a time. I now feel better than I've done for years. I wish I'd done it sooner. This weekend I actually managed to play with a ball in the garden with my six-year-old grandson – all because I stopped smoking. Thank you to everyone in my group at Queen Mary's Hospital.' Barb Wilcox

❯ Excuses for staying a smoker

Here are some reasons smokers commonly give for not quitting – along with the reasons why they don't apply.

Smoking helps me stay thin

Nicotine is an appetite suppressant and increases the rate your body burns calories. When people stop smoking, their metabolism changes and weight gain is possible. This can be managed with nicotine replacement therapy (such as nocotine patches, see Chapter 3) and by watching what you eat. Some people replace cigarettes with comfort eating, which can lead to weight gain – typically 2–3 kg. The risks of smoking far outweigh those from putting on weight. Chapter 9 has plenty of advice on avoiding weight gain after you quit.

Smoking helps me when I'm stressed

The reality is that smokers experience higher levels of stress than non-smokers. After stopping, the level of stress in ex-smokers drops noticeably. For the first few weeks you are likely to experience mood swings and be irritable. There is little evidence that smoking relieves stress – in fact the reverse. Stress and anxiety are reduced rather than increased by giving up smoking. Chapter 7 has advice on coping with stress.

Smoking helps me concentrate

Although many people believe smoking helps them clear their thoughts and concentrate on the task in hand, research shows nicotine does not enhance a smoker's performance level above that of a non-smoker's. This means that when you stop smoking you will be able to focus and concentrate just as well as before.

I feel fit and healthy so there's no rush to stop

Although you may feel fit and healthy, medical tests would probably show evidence of changes in your body caused by smoking. A reduction in lung function, higher blood-fat levels and poorer circulation could demonstrate that you're not as fit as you think. Try taking your pulse before and after you smoke. Notice how fast your heart beats after a cigarette. Imagine this going on in your body 20 plus times a day and you have to ask yourself, how can this be good for me?

I know people who have got cancer after they quit

Stopping smoking at any age increases your life expectancy. Unfortunately, during the years you were a smoker, you've been exposed to toxic chemicals and cancer-causing substances. You cannot wipe out all the damage that may have already occurred. In some people, that damage only becomes apparent in the early years after stopping.

I only smoke cigars

Cigars are not a safe alternative to cigarettes. Switching to cigars from cigarettes gives you the same risk of developing cancer, so don't kid yourself they are better for you. The same is true for pipe smokers and other forms of tobacco.

I've switched to light/low-tar cigarettes

A third of those smoking so-called 'light' or 'low-tar' cigarettes said they chose this type to reduce their health risks. They are no less harmful than other cigarettes. To get the nicotine they need, smokers compensate by taking more or deeper puffs, or by blocking the ventilation holes in the filter. So they take in more tar than they realise. There is no evidence that switching to lower-tar cigarettes reduces the risk of cancer.

People who smoke 'light' cigarettes are half as likely to quit as other smokers. This is due to the false perception that low-tar and low-nicotine cigarettes reduce the risks. The UK banned the terms 'light', 'mild', 'low-tar' on cigarette packs in 2003, because they gave a misleading impression that these products were less harmful than other types.

I only smoke five a day

Moderation is not the answer. Most risks from smoking come with the first few cigarettes of the day. Just one cigarette a day triples the risk of lung cancer, while a five-a-day habit increases a woman's risk of dying of lung cancer fivefold. Those who smoke up to five cigarettes a day are three times more likely to die of heart disease, and more likely to die from all causes, than those who never smoked.

I'm already ill – the damage is done

Most medical treatments work more effectively when someone stops smoking. Being a smoker greatly increases the risk of complications during and after surgery. Smokers are far more likely to have problems and complications with the anaesthetic when they are recovering. Wounds are slower to heal and smokers have a higher chance of chest infection. Stopping weeks, if not months, before surgery is best. If you were able to stop six months before an operation your risk of post-operative complications would be the same as someone who has never smoked. Even stopping three days before having anaesthetic can reduce some of the problems. It allows your blood to get a higher percentage of oxygen circulating, which improves healing and recovery.

I failed last time – I don't want to go through that again

Using a treatment product (Chapter 3) and getting help and support (Chapter 5) can make you up to four times more likely to quit than going cold turkey. Most smokers make several attempts before they break the habit. When you are ready, a good idea is to prioritise your next attempt and make it the most important thing you are doing. The advice in this book will help.

Stopping last time made me feel worse

Withdrawal symptoms can make you feel ill for a few weeks but they pass. Using treatment products will lessen the problems you experience. If you don't stop and become seriously ill because of smoking, you'll have more to cope with than a cough.

There's too much going on right now

There's never going to be a perfect time to stop smoking. Don't put off quitting because of the mythical idea that on the right day it will all be plain sailing. Just choose a date that's likely to be less problematic than most and get on with it. The result is worth it.

An ex-smoker's story

'Some friends were doing a 20-mile charity bike ride and teased me that I was not up to it because I smoked. To prove them wrong I joined in. On the ride I had a few cigarettes to keep me going. I felt very pleased with myself as I'd had no problems keeping up. What I didn't know was that at the end of the ride we were going to visit a hospital and give presents to the children on the cancer ward. I have never felt so bad as when I saw those little children with cancer. They were innocent – but I wasn't. I knew the risk I was taking, but until that moment hadn't thought it through. Suddenly, the truth hit home, I was tempting fate by smoking. I felt such disgust with myself that I never lit up again.' John Hall

---

❯ And finally...

Last, but by no means least, it is getting increasingly difficult to smoke when and where you want. Long gone are the days when you could light up at the cinema, or on the bus or train, or at work. You may have found family and friends don't let you smoke indoors. And from July 2007, smoking will be banned in all public places in the UK.

Think about it. As a smoker, you go through the agony of withdrawal every time you want a cigarette but can't have one. For as long as you smoke, the agony stays the same. From the moment you quit, your withdrawal symptoms get easier, until you no longer suffer at all. Why torture yourself? Convinced? Good! Now turn to the next chapter and start preparing for the moment when you become a non-smoker.

Top tips

- From the moment you quit your body will start to get fitter and healthier.
- Giving up smoking means you'll feel better, sleep better and smell better.
- Once you quit you'll no longer pose a health risk to children.
- After five years your risk of heart attack falls to around half that of a smoker.
- After 10 years your risk of lung cancer falls to around half that of a smoker and your risk of heart attack falls to about the same as someone who has never smoked.

Chapter 2
Preparing To Quit

So, you've decided that the time is right to stop smoking. Well done! There are many more people in the UK who have stopped smoking than are currently smoking – and soon you'll be one of them. You'll gain so much from giving up and put so many problems behind you, you'll wonder why you didn't make this decision long before.

There is no reason why you shouldn't succeed. There is no such thing as being 'too old' or 'too addicted' to quit. You have the power to quit this time, even if you've tried once or even ten times before. You'll find many of the skills you need to call on to give up smoking are the same as those you've used in other areas of your life where you've made significant changes. Having made the decision, you just need to plan how.

⊗ Setting your 'quit date'

The first step is to choose a date to stop smoking. This is your 'quit date'. Setting a 'quit date' is a very important step as it not only helps define the starting point of your stop smoking programme but also confirms your commitment to yourself. If setting a quit date still seems a challenge, don't worry, this chapter is designed to help. The more preparation you put in ahead of time the better, so choose a 'quit date' that gives you enough time to get organised. You are about to set off on a new journey and working out the best route will help you reach your destination successfully.

An ex-smoker's story

'I quit five weeks ago as I'm trying for a baby. I can't say it's easy – pubs are a nightmare – yet it really isn't as bad as I thought it would be. I've joined a gym so on days off I go there to try to distract myself from wanting to smoke. I don't need to smoke, I know that, but I enjoyed smoking. That's the hard thing, to stop something you enjoy. If you are determined enough then anything is possible and I'm very stubborn when I set my mind to something.' Tracy Marshall

Select a day that is likely to be as stress free as possible, or you could be subconsciously setting yourself up to fail. Think about what is going on in your life to help you pick a good day. For example, if you made 'giving up smoking' a new year resolution, it's probably best not to quit on 1st January – wait until the 5th or 6th, when the party season is over and there will be less temptation to smoke.

If you're moving home, consider putting off the quit date until everything is settled and you have a definite date for completion, otherwise the stress of selling up and buying another place might cause a relapse. But once the contracts are signed, the moving-in date would make a good date to stop smoking. Packing and unpacking will keep you busy, so you'll have less free time to smoke. You'll have the incentive of wanting to keep your new home 'smoke free' from the word go, and it will not have the same 'smoking associations' as your old home, so that will make things easier, too.

If you are job hunting, the stress of interviews may encourage you to smoke. But once you start at a new company, you'll have lots of things to learn and fresh faces to meet, and that should keep your mind off the urge to smoke. Plus, new colleagues won't know you as a smoker and you won't link your new workplace with smoking.

Students would probably do best to avoid the exam period of May/June but they could prepare to do it afterwards. Those who have been away at university may be going home to parents who don't know they smoke. It's best if you can get over the worst symptoms, such as being irritable, weepy, or feeling sick, before you see your parents.

If unexpected challenges occur on the day you choose, you can either decide on another day or – as in the examples above – use them to your advantage. There never will be a perfect day to quit smoking, so don't start looking for reasons to put it off. The day you choose will probably be a compromise, but you'll be glad you made the decision.

If you are still not ready to set a quit date, its best to delay your plans. Spending a little longer ensuring you are fully committed is a really good idea and will be much better than having a half-hearted go. You deserve to succeed and are much more likely to achieve your goal when you know the time is right for you.

⟩ Commit to quit

People who put their commitment in writing and tell others what they plan to do are often more successful in achieving their goals than those who don't. They've made up their mind and worked out a strategy to cope with the early days. One approach is to draw up a contract, committing yourself to giving up.

THE
STOP-SMOKING
CONTRACT

I have decided to give up smoking.

I am going to commit myself to the following actions:

I will stop smoking on ....(Date)

After this date I shall never accept another cigarette.

I will inform family, friends and work colleagues of my intention.

After stopping I shall never buy another cigarette.

Signed ....

Witnessed ....

Witnessed ....

Witnessed ....

Nicotine aids or medication?

The next step is to decide how you are going to deal with nicotine withdrawal. Don't ignore this issue. These unpleasant sensations cause many people to return to smoking. Willpower helps but is not always enough on its own. Studies have shown that the best way to stop smoking is with a combination of determination, motivational support and treatment products. Experts recommend nicotine replacement therapy (NRT), such as nicotine patches or gum, or medication such as Zyban to help smokers quit.

NRT gives you back the nicotine you are not getting from smoking. Zyban is a non-nicotine tablet that reduces your craving and eases your symptoms. Such products double your long-term chances of quitting. The National Institute for Health and Clinical Excellence (NICE) is a government body that advises the NHS on treatments. NICE carefully considered the evidence on NRT and Zyban and found both products equally effective in helping smokers quit.

NRT can be bought over the counter from the pharmacist and from some shops. It is also available on prescription. You need to start using NRT the moment you quit. Zyban can only be given on your doctor's prescription as your medical details need to be assessed to ensure the product is suitable for you, so you should discuss it with your GP. Unlike NRT, you start taking Zyban two weeks before your quit date. NRT and Zyban have similar success rates so if you decide on this option it is simply a matter of choosing the one that suits you. NRT and Zyban are discussed in the next chapter. Both are more effective when combined with emotional and behavioural support, such as the NHS Stop Smoking Service (see Chapter 5).

Take the nicotine dependency test

Do you find it difficult not to smoke in situations where you normally would do so?

 Yes   No

Have you tried to stop smoking in the past but found that you could not?

 Yes   No

Answering 'yes' to either of these questions means you are likely to benefit from getting professional advice to help you quit.

How many cigarettes per day do you usually smoke?

	Score
10 or fewer	0
11–20	1
21–30	2
31 or more	3

How soon after you wake do you smoke your first cigarette?

	Score
Within 5 minutes	3
6 –30 minutes	2
31 minutes or more	0

Do you find it difficult to stop smoking in non-smoking areas?

No	0
Yes	1

Which cigarette would you most hate to give up?

First in the morning	1
Other	0

Do you smoke more frequently in the hours after waking than the rest of the day?

No	0
Yes	1

Do you smoke when you are ill in bed for most of the day?

No	0
Yes	1

The numbers added together will give you your dependency score. The higher the number, the greater your need for nicotine replacement therapy.

❯ Changing habits

Habits are created and reinforced over long periods. If you are considering making a change to your smoking, the next step is to look closely at how you have been handling life as a smoker. For many smokers, lighting up is an automatic response to a thought, feeling or external event. Smoking doesn't feel like a separate act but the natural thing to do, no different to eating or speaking. It's a good idea to become aware of your personal triggers and smoking patterns, because there will be times when you find yourself 'automatically' thinking of lighting up, even after you've stopped. Making yourself aware of these stimuli will help you make a successful transition to being a non-smoker.

Tick the times during the day when you are likely to smoke
○ On waking up.
○ To give myself a break.
○ After a meal.
○ When using the telephone.
○ When I need to think.
○ Watching television.
○ When relaxing.

Tick the times when you are likely to smoke more than normal
○ Social events.
○ In confrontational situations.
○ Under personal stress.
○ When working under pressure.
○ When drinking alcohol.
○ Others.

Chapters 6 and 7 will help you find new ways to cope without smoking.

⊘ Need support and advice?

Now you need to decide who you will get to support you. Some people tell everyone they know they have stopped smoking; others wait for their friends to notice. There are no rules on this one, it's up to you, but have at least one phone number handy in case you want to talk to someone. For many people, getting support is a vital part of the process. The NHS can help with advice and treatment options. There are local smoking cessation groups who will give practical tips, and where you will meet other people who are giving up. Together you can give each other emotional support.

The NHS Smoking Helpline 0800 169 0 169 offers a telephone advice service and your local NHS Stop Smoking service runs support groups and one-to-one sessions. Support is covered in more detail in Chapter 5. For a list of international websites and helplines, see page 190.

Carbon monoxide testing

NHS Stop Smoking Services include carbon monoxide (CO) testing as part of the regular meetings. This test gives you a visual demonstration of the presence of damaging levels of carbon monoxide in your expired breath. The technique is simple. You take a deep breath in and hold it for about 15 seconds. You then blow out completely into the monitor, which will give you a reading within seconds. It's a good idea to record this number and do the test again when you have quit smoking. Your new lower reading will be the first proof you have that your body is benefiting when you stop smoking.

Recording your CO readings

Before stopping	
Week One	
Week Two	
Week Three	
Week Four	

An ex-smoker's story

'I wanted to stop this time for several reasons – my health, the cost and because it makes me smell. More and more of my friends were stopping and I started to feel very much in a minority. I felt silly when restaurants made me go outside to smoke. I know that if I don't stop before the complete ban on smoking in public places comes into force, I will be a very angry person when it does. I don't want to become that person and don't want to be forced to sneak cigs in where I can.' Andrea Watson

❯ Think of the money you'll save!

To reinforce your decision to quit, concentrate on all the advantages of giving up smoking. We looked at the health issues in Chapter 1. Now let's look in more detail at the cost. Smoking is an expensive habit and it won't get any cheaper. Just think about all the money you'll save if you quit now. You might be in for a surprise! If you've been buying cigarettes each day you may not realise just how much you've been spending, especially if you include cigarettes in your weekly shop, along with the groceries. Smoking is a very costly habit. A-pack-a-day smoker spends around £40 a week. When you add this up it works out at £2,000 a year. That's how much money you would have available to spend if you gave up now. Of course, if you smoke more than a pack a day you'll save even more!

Work out how much you spend on tobacco each week

Multiply your weekly sum by 52 to find your annual spend:

Each year I spend _____ on tobacco/cigarettes

Think about how long you have been a smoker and try to work out approximately how much money you have spent so far on smoking.

The total amount of money I have spent on smoking is _____

How much more money will you spend if you continue to smoke?

In two years _____

In four years _____

In six years _____

List some things you could you spend this money on

1	
2	
3	
4	
5	

❯ Plan a reward

Rewarding yourself for your efforts is important. After all, who deserves it more? When you are trying to stop smoking you should plan something nice and, thanks to the money you'll save, you will have the money to do so. Many smokers manage to quit simply by focusing on the big reward they've planned for themselves.

List some rewards you could give yourself:

1	
2	
3	
4	
5	

❯ Reasons for stopping smoking

Smokers often need pretty powerful reasons for giving up. These range from negative ones like 'I'm scared of getting cancer,' to positive ones such as 'I want to play football with my children without getting breathless.' There are likely to be many things you don't like about your habit or wish were easier to manage. Here are some reasons people have given for deciding to quit. You may have your own personal reasons for giving up, so add them to the list in the space provided.

Financial reasons

- ☐ Cigarettes are getting expensive.
- ☐
- ☐

Social reasons

- ☐ My partner hates me smoking.
- ☐ I don't want my breath and hair to smell.
- ☐ I hate leaving warm places to go outside to smoke.
- ☐
- ☐

Emotional reasons

- ☐ A friend has just died from smoking, it could have been me. I want to stop before I get ill.
- ☐ Smoking controls me, I want to get back in charge of my life.
- ☐
- ☐

Common sense reasons

- ☐ Socially it's getting harder to smoke.
- ☐ My life insurance cover is higher because I smoke.
- ☐ Most of my friends don't smoke any more.
- ☐ I'd like to set a good example to my kids.
- ☐
- ☐

Personal reasons

☐   I want to start a family.

☐

☐

❯ Get organised

Before you stop smoking it is really important to have a clear
plan of action. If you know what you are going to do from day
one you are less likely to get caught out by an unexpected
problem. To help you, below is a 'quit date' organiser. As you
read through this chapter and the ones that follow, and decide
how you want to give up smoking, you can fill in this page (or
make a copy) to record your plans.

My 'Quit Date' Organiser

My Quit Date is:

I have chosen it because:

The people who are going to support me are:

☐

☐

My emergency 'phone a friend' number/s are:

☐

☐

☐ NHS Smoking Helpline **0800 169 0 169**

These are the rewards/treats I'm giving myself:

After 1 day

After 1 week

After 1 month

After 3 months

At the one year anniversary

Imagination time

Think of some of the bigger treats you could afford with the money you'll save

☐ **A weekend break?**

☐ **New clothes?**

☐ **A holiday?**

☐ **A car?**

☐

☐

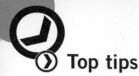

⟩ Top tips

- Choose a 'quit date' that will be as hassle free for you as possible.
- Make a written commitment and tell your friends, family and colleagues.
- List all your reasons for giving up and keep it by you at all times.
- Decide which cigarettes you'll miss most and plan a coping strategy.
- Consider nicotine replacement (e.g. patches or gum) or medication (Zyban).
- Assess your addiction level and decide if you need to seek professional advice.
- Think how much you'll save and plan a reward to buy with the money.

Chapter 3
Managing Nicotine Withdrawal

The pleasurable feelings you get when you smoke come from the nicotine in the cigarettes. Unfortunately, cigarettes also contain tar, which itself contains 4,000 harmful chemical compounds. Along with the carbon monoxide produced by burning tobacco, these tar compounds are what do the damage. They are unwelcome by-products of smoking. To put it bluntly, you smoke for the nicotine but die from the tar.

One of the main reasons stopping smoking is difficult is that your body craves nicotine. This craving makes you feel irritable and anxious and when you quit for the first time the withdrawal symptoms are very strong. Most people find the first few days difficult and you may start to imagine life without smoking will be one long struggle. But if you prepare for these symptoms and decide how to manage them then you won't fall into the trap of thinking that returning to smoking is the only way to 'fix' the problem.

⊘ What is nicotine?

Nicotine is a highly addictive and fast-acting drug. When tobacco smoke is inhaled, nicotine enters the lungs and crosses into the bloodstream, affecting the brain just 7–10 seconds later. Nicotine causes the brain to release chemicals that relax and stimulate you and activate the brain's 'pleasure' centres. Smokers unconsciously adjust the amount they smoke to maintain an optimal level of nicotine in their blood – enough to satisfy the craving but not so much they suffer unwanted side effects like dizziness or nausea.

Over time, the brain gets used to nicotine and you may need to smoke more to get the same feelings of pleasure and relaxation. Reducing the number of cigarettes you smoke or switching to a lower-strength brand just makes you take longer and deeper breaths to get the same amount of nicotine into your body. When you quit smoking, your brain continues to need its daily fix. That is why you get withdrawal symptoms.

Pitfalls of cold turkey

There are over 12 million adult smokers in the UK: 26 per cent of men and 23 per cent of women in the UK smoke. The highest prevalence is in the 20–24 age group, of whom 32 per cent smoke. Despite these large numbers, about 70 per cent of smokers say they would like to give up and about four million smokers try to quit each year. Unfortunately, nicotine is as addictive as heroin or cocaine, which is why there is a very low success rate among those who attempt it unaided, using the 'cold turkey' method.

❯ NRT and Zyban

Quitting doesn't have to be a difficult period of 'cold turkey'. The two recommended options for dealing with withdrawal symptoms are nicotine replacement therapy (NRT) and Zyban. NRT releases controlled amounts of nicotine into the body without the tar, carbon monoxide and other toxins you get from tobacco. Zyban doesn't release nicotine but has a direct effect on the brain that eases withdrawal symptoms. Zyban is discussed in more detail later in this chapter. First we look at NRT.

❯ Understanding Nicotine Replacement

Nicotine replacement therapy (NRT) is much safer and far less addictive than cigarettes. All types of NRT deliver a lower dose of nicotine than you get from cigarettes. It doesn't provide a complete replacement, nor does it eradicate the need for willpower. But it takes the edge off the need to smoke by curbing the cravings and withdrawal symptoms. Using NRT allows you to concentrate on breaking the behavioural side of your smoking habit, such as always lighting up in certain situations.

NRT is not a magic cure but, combined with willpower, it helps you overcome the desire to smoke. Clinical trials show that NRT doubles the chance of success of smokers determined to stop. NRT is available on NHS prescription, from the local NHS Stop Smoking Services and is on sale in many shops.

Some smokers are wary of using NRT products, believing that nicotine itself is harmful. In fact, NRT simply gives your body a small dose of nicotine without the harmful effects of tobacco. Taking a short course of NRT is 99 per cent safer than smoking. It's the other constituents of tobacco that cause the real health damage. NRT helps you gradually reduce your body's addiction by using a low, controlled nicotine dose. People who follow the full 10–12 week course get the best results.

❯ How do I choose the right type for me?

There are currently five types of NRT product available: patches, gum, nasal spray, microtabs, lozenges and inhalator. The way nicotine is delivered and controlled varies between products. This range is wide enough to allow you to find one that will suit your lifestyle. As yet there is little evidence favouring one NRT product over any other. They all seem to have similar success rates, so the choice is a personal and practical one.

❯ Nicotine patches

Nicotine patches are discreet and easy to use and, as a once-a-day solution, are most suitable for smokers who have a regular pattern of smoking. Patches release a steady dose of nicotine into the bloodstream via the skin. The 16-hour patches are worn during the day and taken off at night. The 24-hour patches are worn continuously and are useful for people who experience early morning cravings.

Patches should be applied to a relatively hairless part of the body such as the upper arm. The patch site must be changed daily – never put it on the same place two days running. You shouldn't smoke while the patch is on. The recommended time for using a patch is 12 weeks. Patches are available in three strengths to allow users to step down the dose when they feel ready. In general, people who smoke 10 cigarettes or more a day should start with the highest dose patch.

Occasionally, patches can cause local skin irritation, although this usually passes after a few days. A week's supply of patches costs in the region of £15. You can also ask your GP to provide them on prescription.

❯ Nicotine gum

Nicotine gum comes in a variety of flavours and lets you control your nicotine dose yourself. Learning to use the gum properly is important. You chew it gently until you notice the flavour coating your mouth. Then you stop chewing and 'park' the gum in your cheek, allowing the nicotine that's just been released to be absorbed through the lining of the mouth. When the taste has faded, the gum is chewed again and re-parked any nicotine that is swallowed cannot be absorbed into your bloodstream and may cause unpleasant side effects.

The 2 mg gum is effective for those who smoke 20 cigarettes or fewer per day and the 4 mg is for those who smoke more than 20 per day. Most people use 10–15 pieces of gum daily for at least the first 12 weeks and gradually reduce the number of pieces chewed.

❯ Nicotine nasal spray

Nicotine nasal spray is the strongest form of NRT available. The nicotine is in solution in a small bottle. You tip your head back slightly and insert the nozzle into the nostril. The bottom of the container is pressed to administer a single spray. Repeat for each nostril.

You'll need one or two doses per hour for the first eight weeks and then you reduce the dosage over the next four weeks. The nasal spray gives rapid relief from cravings and is especially suitable for heavy and highly addicted smokers as it is absorbed faster than any other NRT. It is recommended for those who smoke more than 20 cigarettes per day and/or those who light up within 30 minutes of waking. The spray can cause local irritant effects such as runny nose, sneezing, throat irritation. These side effects should lessen with use, usually after a few days. It's important to remember that the irritation will stop soon so try to persevere.

❯ Nicotine microtab

The microtab is a small, white tablet that you put under your tongue and leave in place. As it slowly dissolves, nicotine is gradually absorbed through the lining of the mouth. The micro tab should be taken for at least 12 weeks, over which time the amount used can be gradually reduced. It should not be sucked, chewed or swallowed as this stops the absorption of nicotine.

❯ Nicotine lozenge

The lozenge is like a sweet that you let dissolve slowly in your mouth. It delivers the nicotine to you in a similar way to the microtab.

❯ Nicotine inhalator

The inhalator is a plastic device shaped like a cigarette with a nicotine cartridge fitted into it. Sucking on the mouthpiece, like a cigarette, releases nicotine vapour. This gets absorbed through your mouth and throat and is not inhaled into the lungs. Because it's held like a cigarette, it's suitable for people who miss the habit of holding and handling a cigarette. To get the most from the inhalator it's important to follow the 12-week programme. From 6 to 12 cartridges should be used each day for the first 8 weeks and then the numbers should be reduced over the next 4 weeks. However, the number needed often depends on how many cigarettes you are used to smoking.

This graph shows the levels of nicotine taken in by smoking cigarettes compared to nicotine replacement therapy products[1]:

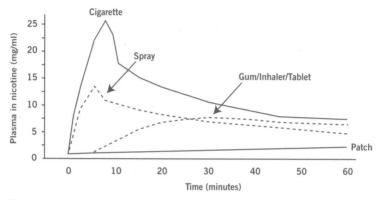

❯ Frequently asked questions

Can I get addicted to NRT?

You are unlikely to get addicted to NRT as the dose is smaller. Unlike cigarettes, which deliver nicotine in an immediate and high dose, delivery from NRT is slower and more controlled. The level of immediate satisfaction is not the same. NRT releases nicotine at a constant rate, causing less fluctuation in nicotine levels. This helps control the addiction to cigarettes while allowing you to wean yourself off nicotine.

Even if you end up using NRT over a longer time than recommended, the risk is small compared to the much greater risks of continuing to smoke. It is important to follow the instructions and gradually reduce the amount of NRT you use after 8 to 12 weeks.

1 Graph reproduced from *Nicotine Addiction in Britain* courtesy of the Royal College of Physicians, adapted from Russell, MAH: 'Nicotine Intake and its Regulation by Smokers' in *Tobacco Smoking & Nicotine: A Neurobiological Approach*. WR Martin, GRV Loon, ET Iwamoto and L Davis, Plenum Publishing Corporation, New York (1987)

Is nicotine replacement harmful?

Nicotine has not been found to cause cancer or be directly harmful in any other way. It is the tar and other toxins in tobacco that cause disease. NRT is much safer than many people realise.

Will NRT keep me craving nicotine?

No, the amount from NRT that you get is just enough to help you beat the craving to smoke but not enough to keep you addicted. Manufacturers recommend you follow the step-down plan, to learn to reduce your nicotine intake until you no longer need it. NRT is not a replacement for willpower but helps you manage withdrawal symptoms. The best way to use NRT is to combine it with structured support, the sort that can be obtained from you local NHS Stop Smoking Service (see Chapter 5).

Are there any side effects with NRT?

All medicines have the potential to cause side effects. Those experienced with NRT are not serious and are similar to the known actions of nicotine and would be experienced by a smoker who has smoked rapidly or more frequently than they normally did.

How long does a course of NRT last?

A full course of NRT lasts 12 weeks. It is important that smokers know how to use the products properly. One of the most common problems with NRT is that people fail to use enough of it, for long enough, to enable them to quit successfully and stay stopped. Occasionally, if a smoker has real concerns about relapse they may wish to remain on the product for a few more weeks, which can be allowed.

How do I know which dose to use?

NRT isn't meant to give you the same feelings as smoking. Smokers who use more than 15 cigarettes a day usually start on the highest strength NRT and gradually wean themselves off it over the 12-week course. Ideally they would have eight weeks on full strength, then two weeks on middle strength and finally two weeks on lowest strength. In practice, smokers decide for themselves when they feel ready to reduce the strength of NRT they are using. If they use too much NRT they may feel nauseated and dizzy. Reducing the dose eliminates these symptoms.

Are NRT products expensive?

You can get NRT on prescription from your doctor or via your local NHS Stop Smoking Service. For details, call the NHS Smoking Helpline on 0800 169 0 169. Even if you buy NRT products over the counter, this is much cheaper than continuing to smoke. At today's rates, a 20-a-day smoker will spend more than £2,000 a year on tobacco.

Is NRT safe if I have heart disease?

Stopping smoking is the most important thing someone can do to slow the progression of the disease. Using NRT to quit outweighs any risks there might be with the product.

Can I use NRT if I'm pregnant?

If you have found that you cannot give up smoking during your pregnancy, you can consider using NRT. The evidence is that continuing to smoke is far more harmful for pregnant and breastfeeding women than using NRT. If you are concerned, speak to your midwife or doctor about your specific circumstances.

Can I use NRT if I'm under 16?

NRT is as well tolerated by teenagers as by adults and safer than smoking. There is no evidence to show adolescents misuse or abuse NRT. The recommended maximum course for a teenager is 12 weeks, after which they should seek medical advice before continuing.

I've still got some symptoms despite using NRT?

If you still have cravings or other physical symptoms while using NRT, you may need to increase the dose. Sometimes it can take a few days to work out the exact level of nicotine your body needs to feel comfortable and you may need to experiment to get it just right.

Is it safe to use two types of NRT together?

Some smokers benefit from using two types of NRT simultaneously, such as a patch with the gum, inhalator, nasal spray or micro tab. This provides a constant release of nicotine via the patch and, if cravings still arise, allows you to top up your nicotine level with an oral preparation. It's worth considering this option if you were previously unsuccessful using one type only, for example, if you were irritable, moody or short-tempered.

In practice, many people discover through trial and error what type of NRT works best for them. It's always worth talking to a healthcare professional if you are worried or experiencing symptoms. As well as being a sign of nicotine withdrawal, symptoms might indicate that you haven't found a way to replace the role cigarettes play in your life.

Champix (Varenicline)

Champix is a new non-nicotine drug which has been shown to have a favourable safety profile. Champix works by relieving the craving and withdrawal symptoms associated with stopping smoking. It blocks nicotine from working, so if the smoker slips and has a cigarette, the pleasure and satisfaction of smoking will be reduced with less risk of returning to smoking.

Champix is taken in tablet form and needs to be prescribed by a doctor. The treatment course is twelve weeks but this can be doubled to increase the smoker's chance of staying smoke free. In two clinical trials, 44 per cent of smokers quit smoking by the end of 12 weeks, and a year later around 1 in 5 still didn't smoke.

Can I cut down before I stop smoking?

The only way to reduce the risks from smoking is to stop completely. If you cannot do this, you can use NRT while cutting down. Research shows that for people who cannot quit suddenly, a gradual approach using nicotine replacement products significantly increases their chances of successfully stopping.

Smokers trying this method can also use two forms of NRT at the same time – the gum and inhalator – to reduce the number of cigarettes they smoke as a step towards stopping completely. Smokers who try this route are expected to cut down their cigarette consumption over six to nine months, while using nicotine replacement products to reduce cravings.

NRT boosts nicotine levels, making it easier to smoke fewer cigarettes, which in turn means the smoker inhales fewer toxins. By reducing their reliance on cigarettes for their nicotine intake, some smokers can then stop smoking completely.

This method is suitable for smokers who are not ready to stop, or do not want to stop but want to cut down with a view to stopping. Stopping totally remains the ideal but this method offers a useful introduction to NRT before giving up.

How to use the cutting down method

You should use the NRT gum or inhaler between cigarettes whenever you experience an urge to smoke. The aim is to extend your smoke-free intervals and reduce your smoking as much as possible.

Step 1: (0–6 weeks) – Start cutting down

- Set a target for the number of cigarettes per day to cut down and a date to achieve it by – a 50 per cent reduction gives the best results.
- Try to replace every second cigarette with NRT.
- Use the gum or inhalator as required to manage cravings.
- Seek professional advice if you find cutting down hard.

Step 2: (6 weeks to 6 months) – Continue cutting down

- Continue to cut down cigarettes using gum.
- The goal is to stop smoking completely by six months.
- Seek professional advice if still smoking at nine months.

Step 3: (within 9 months) – Stop smoking

- Stop all cigarettes and continue to use gum or inhalator to relieve cravings.

Step 4: (within 12 months) – *Stop NRT*

- Gradually cut down use of the gum or inhalator, then stop completely within three months of stopping smoking.

⊗ Understanding Zyban

Zyban is the trade name for bupropion hydrochloride, a prescription-only medicine originally prescribed as an antidepressant. It is a non-nicotine tablet that reduces the desire to smoke and so eases withdrawal symptoms. It is very effective and has helped approximately one in five people who take it to give up smoking. Worldwide it has helped millions of smokers to stop.

Its ability to help smokers quit was found by chance when patients reported they had lost their desire to smoke. It is not known exactly how Zyban works, but it's thought to interrupt the areas of the brain that are associated with addiction and the pleasurable effects of nicotine. In other words, it suppresses the part of the brain that gives the smoker a nicotine buzz. This reduces the craving to smoke and dampens the physical symptoms of nicotine withdrawal, such as anxiety, sweating and irritability.

The advantages of Zyban

Zyban has been shown to double a smoker's chances of successfully quitting when compared to using willpower alone. A course lasts two months, and you should be prepared to stop smoking by the second week of the course. The drug helps you because you no longer get the 'hit' when you smoke. People start on one tablet a day for six days and then increase this to two tablets a day.

The disadvantages of Zyban

Zyban is only available on prescription and is not suitable for everyone, so you must talk through your full medical history with your doctor before starting a course. You should not use Zyban if you are pregnant or breastfeeding, and you must take extra care when driving. Zyban is not suitable for people with a history of blackouts, fits, head injury or a brain tumour, or for those withdrawing from high alcohol intake or tranquilliser/ antidepressant-type drugs. Care must also be taken if you are on some other types of medicines. As with all drugs, there is a risk of side-effects. Some users report unpleasant symptoms such as nausea, headaches, dry mouth and blurred vision.

❯ Frequently asked questions

When was Zyban first used?

This drug has been used extensively in the USA as an antidepressant for a number of years under the trade name Wellbutrin.

What is the success rate?

Research has confirmed that it is an effective treatment for tobacco dependence. In a clinical trial, it was found that 12 months after finishing the course of Zyban, 23 per cent of users had remained smoke free.

What are the risks of taking Zyban?

Zyban was the subject of scare stories and negative publicity such as 'Anti-smoking drug deaths' and confidence in the product dropped, but the dangers of continuing to smoke are far, far greater. The National Institute for Health and Clinical Excellence (NICE) issued guidance confirming the confidence of the regulators in Zyban. They state that, along with NRT, Zyban is one of the best treatments available for stopping smoking. However, it is possible to buy Zyban abroad without a prescription and use it unsupervised. This is dangerous. Always see your GP for a prescription to ensure Zyban is suitable and safe with regard to your own particular medical history.

An ex-smoker's story

'I have smoked since I was 15. I've tried to stop quite a few times over the years – I would guess about 10 times. I can't give you a good reason for my relapses but I can say that I remember having a drink in my hand when I did. So I can only associate relapsing with alcohol. I decided to check out Zyban and talked to my doctor. He said he would prescribe it if I wanted to give it a go. It made me feel rather sickly at first but I feel fine now. I was told to take it for two weeks before I stopped smoking. On my

quit date I was surprised that I didn't think about smoking at all. I had tried NRT patches, inhalators and tablets and nothing worked – though maybe that was down to my lack of determination! I have lots of people supporting me. I think my biggest challenge will be going on a night out with friends and not smoking. I am surprised and happy that I don't even think about cigarettes. On the odd occasion that I do think about smoking, I reason why I want it and what good it will do me and that talks me out of the temptation.' Andrea Watson

❯ Treatment planner

NRT and Zyban work best as part of an overall NHS Stop Smoking Service support programme. To help you work out which NHS-recommended treatment method will suit you and your lifestyle best, reread all the options and then fill in the treatment planner below.

Are there health problems that may rule out an NRT product?

For example, if you suffer from psoriasis or eczema this may preclude wearing a patch. If you have sore gums/loose teeth or wear dentures this could make using a gum more difficult.

Yes (give details)

No

Do you have any work/lifestyle restrictions?

For example, chewing gum may be prohibited by some employers.

Yes (give details)

No

Have your tried NRT before?

Yes (give details)

No

List any previous types of treatment you have used

- ☐
- ☐
- ☐
- ☐

Has your doctor ruled out Zyban in your case?

Yes (give details)

No

Have your tried Zyban before?

Yes (give details)

No

What medication/ treatment worked for you before?

- ☐
- ☐
- ☐

If you had no success with NRT or Zyban in the past, why do you think this was?

- ☐
- ☐
- ☐

Top tips

- NRT or Zyban doubles your chance of giving up smoking.
- NRT and Zyban help reduce cravings and withdrawal symptoms.
- NRT and Zyban are safer than smoking.
- NRT provides nicotine in a way that is slower and less satisfying, but safer than cigarettes.
- NRT doesn't provide a complete replacement for cigarettes.
- NRT doesn't contain tar, toxic chemicals and carbon monoxide like tobacco smoke.
- NRT does not cause cancer or long-term addiction.
- NRT is not a magic cure but can help a smoker who is determined to stop.
- NRT can be used by patients with heart and circulatory disease.
- NRT can be used by regular smokers aged 12 and over.
- NRT can be used by pregnant smokers under medical supervision.
- More than one form of NRT can be used together.
- NRT can be prescribed for up to nine months.
- NRT can be used while still smoking to reduce consumption before your quit date.
- Zyban is as effective as NRT.
- Zyban suppresses withdrawal symptoms but does not replace nicotine.
- Zyban is only available on prescription from your doctor.
- Zyban is unsuitable if you are pregnant or breastfeeding and can cause side effects.
- Zyban may be unsuitable if you have a medical condition – your doctor will advise.

Chapter 4
Alternative Treatment Methods

There are other methods you can use to help you stop smoking in addition to, or instead of, the methods already discussed. The most widely used alternative methods are acupuncture, cold turkey, complementary therapies, cutting down and hypnotherapy.

Some people find them helpful to stop smoking. However, these methods are not tested in the same way as other treatments described in this book and it's not possible to compare the results to treatments that have undergone rigorous clinical trials. If you decide to choose an alternative therapy, please make sure that the practitioner you use is qualified with the relevant professional body.

⊗ Acupuncture

Acupuncture is a traditional Chinese therapy in which sharp needles are inserted into special 'acupoints' controlling the body's energy channels. The process is not painful and clients are left to relax for half an hour or so. The needles are then removed, except for two tiny ones that remain in the ear. The client is advised to touch an ear lobe when a craving comes on, and this helps the feeling pass. There are no clinical tests to prove the effectiveness of acupuncture in helping smokers quit, but some have found it valuable.

⊗ Aversion therapy

Aversive techniques are based on the principles of 'classical conditioning' in which the behaviour a person wants to change is paired with a bad experience. For example, smokers might try rapid smoking, where cigarettes are smoked quickly one after another. This makes smokers associate their habit with something unpleasant and so, in theory, are more likely to quit. It has been tried with smokers and produced modest results, but there isn't enough evidence to show whether it works or not.

An ex-smoker's story

'I gave up when I had a cold. I bought lots of gum, sweets, fruit, and veg to chew. My treat was malt whiskey. I refused invitations to spend weekends with smokers. I decided to donate the money I was saving to charity, so felt obliged to continue. My pharmacist was great and checked my CO levels. I took it seriously this time and have been successful.' Harry Spencer-Smith

---

⟩ Bioresonance therapy

Practitioners claim this is a painless and holistic method of dealing with the hidden causes of disease and ill health. It works by assessing and normalising energetic imbalances. It is based on the theory that all matter, living and inert, resonates at specific electromagnetic frequencies. Toxic substances such as infections, chemicals and heavy metals alter the body's 'normal' pattern. Proponents say that removing toxic frequencies with bioresonance will modify and correct subtle energy patterns, helping the body to return to its 'normal' healthy status. Its role in helping people stop smoking is unproven.

⟩ Cold turkey

Stopping without any kind of aid is known as going 'cold turkey'. Although physical symptoms can be more extreme in the early few days, they fade away within the first two or three weeks. Most people first try to give up smoking using this method and some succeed – although a high proportion relapse within 12 months of their quit date. Unaided attempts to stop smoking have the least chance of success.

An ex-smoker's story

'I had smoked pretty much full time since I was 16 and only gave up while I was pregnant with my daughter, but that was purely for the baby's health rather than any consideration for my own. Unfortunately, as soon as I finished breastfeeding, the urge to smoke won through again. I don't know why I ever took up smoking; I lost my mother to cancer at the age of 12. She was only 47 and I know her smoking habit was almost certainly related to her death. Even this did not stop me from smoking. I had tried to give up many times and failed. I think what finally made me wake up was a bad persistent cough, something I had never experienced before. It got to the point where I couldn't hold a conversation or even breathe in sometimes without a coughing fit. I got scared and wondered if I had a serious lung disease. It made me realise that I had abused my body for half of my life, and that my body is not as young as it was and won't just keep bouncing back anymore. So I threw my cigarettes away. I decided to go cold turkey, as I have used patches in the past and found that as soon as I tailed them off my cravings came back. I did buy some nicotine gum for emergencies, and would highly recommend it as an instant fix during a craving. It has been really hard and I have had one or two falls off the wagon. However, my motivation is my daughter as I don't want her to lose her mother at a young age as I did. I feel a real sense of purpose on a purely personal level and am proud I've managed to quit and just don't want to jeopardise anything.' Victoria Micklewright

❯ Complementary therapies

Many complementary therapies can help with different aspects of stopping smoking. For example, having an aromatherapy or massage treatment can help you relax. Qualified herbalists and homeopathy practitioners may be able to prescribe remedies that offer symptom relief. The British Complementary Medicine Association provides information about different therapies and can suggest approved therapists in your area. There is no clinical evidence to support the effectiveness of these techniques for smokers who want to quit, but many have found them beneficial.

⟩ Glucose

Taking glucose in the first weeks when you stop smoking may help reduce the severity of the cravings to smoke. Glucose taken in the form of oral dextrose tablets is a very easy substance for the body to absorb and convert into energy. A few minutes after eating a glucose tablet, your blood sugars rise and you won't have to handle the urge to eat. Glucose has been shown to stop the hunger pains and ease nicotine withdrawal.

Glucose may also help because of its effect on the brain chemical serotonin, which is associated with feeling happy and contented. It is known there is a relationship between blood-sugar levels and serotonin in the brain and that low blood-sugar levels can affect mood. Glucose may ease the side effects you get in the first few days after you quit, such as headache, bad moods or difficulty concentrating.

Bear in mind that glucose tablets can be bad for dental health. You'll need to brush and floss your teeth more often than usual and it may help to neutralise the higher acidity levels if you drink some milk or chew a small piece of cheese after eating glucose. People who are diabetic should check with their GP before considering this option.

An ex-smoker's story

'Chewing sugar-free gum helped. I was eating too many sweets to start with. I hate to admit it but swearing a lot seemed to get me through some of the worst times. This is from someone who generally does not swear! My advice to others is to take it one day at a time and be pleased with yourself every day that you have even stopped.' Pat Stocking

---

❯ Private groups and clinics

Smokers who are motivated to quit the habit may benefit from attending private stop-smoking support groups. These offer similar programmes to those run by the National Health Service and charities but with additional services provided. Private clinics can be expensive, so make sure you know the total cost before you sign up. Be cautious about the claims of high success rates made by some private clinics.

❯ Herbal cigarettes

Some herbal cigarettes are suggested as an aid to quit smoking. They contain no nicotine or tobacco, but are smoked in the usual way. However, 'vegetable-based' cigarettes produce a similar level of carbon monoxide to that of tobacco-based cigarettes. This can be a potential health hazard and studies have found no benefit in using this product. Herbal cigarettes also produce significant levels of tar. Another problem is that lighting up a herbal cigarette keeps you hooked on the habit of smoking.

❯ Hypnotherapy

Although nicotine is a physically addictive drug, smoking has many psychological associations. Hypnotherapy tries to alter the mind's dependence on smoking as a habit. The treatment can also help you to relax when you get the desire to smoke and may strengthen your determination to quit. Some people find that hypnotherapy does help them to stop, although it is not a clinically proven method.

> **An ex-smoker's story**
> *'My main reason for quitting was because I suffered from a nasty cough. Every morning I used to spend 15 minutes trying to get my lungs into working order! I started to experience shortness of breath and this really scared me. Another reason, and if I'm honest this was the big motivator for me, was my friend offered to give me one of her beautiful kittens. However she refused to let me have*

him until I stopped smoking. She explained that cats don't like smoke and if I was smoking indoors it would cause the kitten to suffer. I was convinced after that and dumped the habit.' Karina White

❯ Laser treatment

This is a new treatment developed by a former smoker. It uses a painless, low-powered laser to stimulate energy points on the body, rather like acupuncture. This stimulates the production of endorphins – the body's natural pain relief chemicals – and, theoretically, relieves nicotine cravings. There are no clinical tests to prove the effectiveness of laser treatment in helping people give up.

❯ Nicogel

This gel product is sold as a form of nicotine replacement therapy. It is said to contain extracts of tobacco plant (*Nicotiana spp.*) and satisfy the craving for nicotine. It is claimed that it takes less than one minute for the active ingredients in the gel to reach the brain and the effects last for two to four hours. Experts, however, point out that there is no clinical evidence of effectiveness and no way to measure the amount of nicotine that is absorbed when using the product.

❯ NicoBloc

NicoBloc is a stop smoking aid to help users slowly wean themselves off nicotine. It is said to help smokers by progressively reducing the amount of nicotine they inhale. NicoBloc comes as drops of liquid that are applied to the filter of the cigarette immediately before smoking. It works by trapping the nicotine and tar in the filter and so preventing them entering the body. Smokers use it over a six-week period before their planned stop date to help them prepare to stop completely. This is not an NHS recommended treatment as there is no clinical evidence of effectiveness.

⊘ Nicobrevin

Nicobrevin comes as capsules of menthyl valerate (a mild sedative), quinine (a mild appetite suppressant), camphor and eucalyptus (to reduce mucus secretion and accumulation) and is available without prescription. There is no evidence of long-term success. It should not be used in pregnancy.

⊘ Top tips

- Some smokers have found alternative methods can help them quit – although there is little scientific proof to back this up.
- Acupuncture may aid relaxation as well as easing withdrawal symptoms.
- Hypnotherapy can help smokers manage psychological dependence on smoking.
- Other complementary methods that offer symptom relief include aromatherapy, massage, herbalism and homeopathy.
- Glucose tablets can reduce nicotine cravings – but take extra care over dental hygiene.
- Check that the practitioner you use is qualified with the relevant professional body.
- Giving up unaided – cold turkey – has a low success rate.

Chapter 5
Support And Advice To Help You Quit

Anti-withdrawal aids such as NRT and Zyban will help you manage the cravings, but they can't give you the additional support and encouragement that help many smokers give up. For that you will need other people. Some smokers decide to go it alone, which is fine, but most people find they benefit from the support of others. Having supportive friends, relatives and colleagues is fantastic. But it can be even more beneficial to use a planned support system involving trained specialists and advisers.

NHS Stop Smoking Services provide advice and support to bolster a smoker's attempts to quit smoking. And there are many other services available, including specialist services to help pregnant women and teenagers stop, and many businesses now have workplace programmes to encourage their employees to quit.

⊙ NHS Stop Smoking Services

NHS Stop Smoking Services have been highly successful. Research shows that smokers are up to four times more likely to give up successfully if they use their local NHS Stop Smoking Services, combined with nicotine replacement therapy, rather than going it alone and relying on willpower. Around 15 per cent of smokers who set a quit date with the NHS services can be expected to remain non-smokers after a year. More than 300,000 smokers kicked the habit after receiving help from NHS Stop Smoking Services in 2005.

An ex-smoker's story

'I gave up so I could enjoy the freedom, better health and also the wealth. The best decision I made was to join a group – I got excellent support, advice and tips. I got my partner to put my patches on for me if he got up first. It was important to persevere with the symptoms in the first few weeks because they do pass. I got absorbed in programmes on the telly, as I found they took my mind off it.' C. James

What is available for people who smoke?

There are a number of ways to find out about local services and advisers. The NHS Smoking Helpline and website can provide details of local services. Smokers can telephone the service directly to book themselves an appointment or obtain details of a local community adviser (often a local pharmacist). GPs' surgeries and clinics and other health professionals may have their own advisers or can refer patients to local services. Smokers wishing to quit can also contact NHS Direct or ask their local pharmacist about NHS Stop Smoking Services.

Publications

A range of self-help materials are available that provide information and advice on stopping smoking, covering everything from the physical side effects to details about health problems and smoking-related diseases. You can download some of the most popular resources, or order from the full range of resources free via the website www.givingupsmoking.co.uk, or phone the NHS Smoking Helpline on 0800 169 0 169.

'Together' programme

'Together' is a free programme provided by the NHS Stop Smoking Support Team that is designed to help you stop smoking. It is the first such programme of its kind in the UK. It is compiled using medical research and insights from ex-smokers. Through the 'Together' programme, the NHS Stop

Smoking Support Team is with you each step of the way, providing practical help and advice at each stage of the 'giving up' process.

To join 'Together' simply decide on a quit date and register by calling the NHS Smoking Helpline on 0800 169 0 169, quoting 'Together'. You can call the Helpline at any time throughout the programme and speak to a specialist advisor, quoting 'Together'. You can also join the programme by logging on to www.givingupsmoking.co.uk/together.

The support offered by the 'Together' programme includes practical help and advice in the form of information packs sent to your home, emails, phone calls and text messages. When you register, you'll receive advance information to help you prepare:

O **Before your quit date, they'll write to you with help and advice on how to prepare.**

O **Close to your quit date, they give help and advice to get you through your first month.**

O **After the first month, they check to see how you're coping and give encouragement and reassurance.**

O **After three months, they write to you with advice on maintaining your new non-smoking status, or provide further help if you're still trying.**

O **If you choose, they can provide extra support and advice by phone, email and text.**

The 'Together' team can also refer you to your local NHS Stop Smoking Services, where you can arrange to meet a specialist adviser face to face or join a group of fellow smokers who are trying to quit (see below).

NHS Smoking Helpline
The Helpline is open from 7 a.m. to 11 p.m. every day for information requests and referrals, with unlimited access to trained advisers giving one-to-one advice and support. When you phone the Helpline, a friendly adviser will offer confidential

support and advice, or just listen to you. Advisers can also send callers a free 'Giving up for life' booklet, packed with practical tips and advice for giving up, key smoking facts and real-life stories.

Since its launch, the Helpline has received over one million calls. A year after first calling the NHS Smoking Helpline, nearly a quarter of callers said they had successfully given up and were still not smoking. NHS Smoking Helpline advisers can refer callers to a local NHS Stop Smoking Service offering free, ongoing face-to-face support and advice near their own home.

An ex-smoker's story

'I had never used NRT when I tried to stop smoking before. I think my success owes a lot to patches and the inhalator. I also went to a smoking cessation group who gave me lots of practical tips as well as emotional support. Knowing that other people were going through the same things as me, like feeling extremely irritated, helped – it didn't stop me feeling as irritated – but it made me feel normal and I felt able to be open with people about my moods. I tell other people who want to stop smoking, if you can, go to a smoking cessation group as the practical and emotional support is fantastic. I think everyone who's trying to stop should give NRT a try – I think it really works.' Claire Walker

NHS Pregnancy Smoking Helpline

For those worried about smoking during pregnancy (including the partners, friends and family of pregnant women), the NHS Pregnancy Smoking Helpline 0800 169 9 169 offers specialist help and advice on stopping smoking during pregnancy. Included in this service is a dedicated call-back programme, which offers callers periodic follow-up calls during pregnancy and also post-natal. Lines are open daily from 12 noon to 9 p.m.

NHS Asian Tobacco Helpline

The NHS Asian Tobacco Helpline provides advice and support for people speaking the following languages: Urdu, Punjabi, Hindi, Gujurati and Bengali. Specialist advisers can provide confidential advice and tips on giving up smoking or chewing tobacco and/or tobacco paan. Lines are open every Tuesday from 1 p.m. to 9 p.m.

Service for hearing impaired

If you are deaf or hard of hearing, you can use the textphone on 0800 169 0 171.

Behind the scenes at the NHS Smoking Helpline

Up to 12 advisors work at the NHS Smoking Helpline at any one time offering tailored, flexible and personal advice. Alexia Paterson has worked on the Helpline for many years and dealt with all forms of enquires. She explains what happens:

'We start by giving our name and establishing what a caller needs from the service. As the conversation develops, we get a picture of the caller's smoking history. Picking up the phone and talking to a stranger can be a big step. Some people are nervous as they think they're going to be judged. They are always pleasantly surprised by our positive and friendly approach. We explain we can send them out general information, refer them to local NHS Stop Smoking Services, and give advice on the treatments available to help them cope with the nicotine withdrawal symptoms. If callers want immediate help, we ask about their daily pattern of smoking and reasons for wanting to stop and we encourage them to join a group run by their local stop smoking service.

'When hard-hitting adverts about smoking are running on TV we get thousands of extra calls. People get upset by seeing real smokers who have become ill and can be scared of it happening to them. These adverts are definitely bringing home the dangers of smoking. For some, this will be the first time they have ever considered

stopping. We don't have set speeches, as every caller is different. We tailor our advice according to their circumstances. People can call as often as they like and we encourage them to keep in touch with us. After we have helped them stop smoking, many people call to let us know how they are getting on.'

⊘ Local stop smoking services

All the support people need to stop smoking is available through a range of locally based services offered free by the NHS. Most services offer both group support and individual help. Your adviser will tell you all about treatment options. Some advisers can also provide nicotine replacement therapy and Zyban on prescription. Others can help you get this medication from your GP. You don't have to quit on your first meeting – your adviser will tailor a help programme to suit your individual needs.

There are over 170 established local NHS Stop Smoking Services throughout England. Scotland and Wales have similar systems in place. Smokers meet advisers individually or as part of a group. According to which stop smoking service you visit, a group course can run for from five to seven weeks. Smokers join while they are still smoking and typically spend the first two sessions preparing to give up in the third week.

An ex-smoker's story

'Having smoked for 53 years and suffered from cancer of the vocal cords, which thankfully has now been successfully treated, I had tried several times to stop smoking but failed. But when two of my grandchildren said, "Granddad, stop smoking, we don't want you to die," I became determined to give up, so I signed up for the smoking cessation clinic which I found very helpful and have not smoked since my quit day. I can now breathe easier, taste of food has improved and as expected, I have more cash in the pocket.' Anthony Mills

Stop smoking support groups

Support groups are run by health professionals with special training to help smokers quit. Most groups meet for an hour or two a week for six or seven weeks. Group size varies but are usually large enough to compensate for the drop out that can naturally occur to ensure the remaining clients are not affected. As well as benefiting from the support offered by the adviser, support groups allow you to share experiences and tips with fellow quitters. And you won't be left to manage on your own once the meetings end. Many areas run monthly relapse prevention meetings, or regular drop-in sessions.

Behind the scenes at a stop smoking support group

Jo Woodvine is an NHS Smoking Cessation Facilitator for Bexley Stop Smoking Service. She explains how she runs her groups:

'In Bexley, group support can be obtained by joining one of our free six-week stop-smoking clinics. We book up to a maximum of 30 people onto our rolling programme of courses. The group members attend for an hour a week at a local hospital. No one is asked to stop smoking until the second week of the course, when everyone stops at the same time. This is a very powerful and effective way to stop smoking as everybody is at the same stage and can empathise with other group members as they make the change from smoker to non-smoker. Our clinics are extremely popular and successful with usually at least 8 out of 10 people attending managing to quit by the end of the 6-week programme. Some groups have had 100 per cent success rates at the end of the programme.'

⟩ A stop smoking support group

The programme offered by support groups may vary slightly from group to group. But the one at Bexley is typical of many and gives an idea of the service provided.

Week one

The first week is an information/advice session. As soon as new group members arrive they have a carbon monoxide reading taken, for use as a comparison when they stop smoking altogether. The adviser explains what carbon monoxide does to the body and the immediate effect on the reading once they stop. Group members are asked to say why they want to quit and to write down their reasons when they leave the session. They are shown the range of NRT products available and given a letter to take to their GP to obtain NRT on prescription. Members are encouraged to think about what they will do with their time once they stop smoking and about making changes to their routines to make it easier to give up.

Week two

This includes the 'quit day' for the whole group. Members are given reassurance that they can stop smoking. Advisers check that members have chosen an NRT product and can use it efficiently and explain about possible withdrawal symptoms. Staff stress the importance of total abstinence during the coming weeks and ask everyone to choose a 'support buddy' from the group. The buddies phone each other to give encouragement and support – especially during the first seven-day period. Advisers also follow up anyone who fails to show up the following week to find out how they have fared.

Week three

New carbon monoxide readings are taken to monitor level of improvement. Members talk about their first smoking-free week and say whether they have kept in contact with their 'support buddy'. They explain how they dealt with the urge to smoke and say whether they smoked during this first week. They are given advice, such as how to cope around smokers in social settings, and the session ends with everyone promising not to smoke for a further week.

Week four

More carbon monoxide readings are taken and members give progress reports on the past week. They discuss the best and worst things about not smoking, as well as any triggers that might tempt them to start again, and talk about the cost of smoking. They also discuss how to manage cravings, stress and withdrawal symptoms. Group participation is encouraged.

Week five

Once again, carbon monoxide readings are taken and progress reports given, and the discussion turns to how members are using NRT, handling risky situations and the benefits of positive thinking. By now, NRT should have eased the addictive side of smoking. So now members focus on the psychological aspects. Members discuss the changes they have made to replace their smoking rituals, and talk about the benefits of not smoking and any improvements they have noticed in their health.

Week six

For group members who have stayed smoking free, it's time to celebrate! They receive a certificate and huge applause. Members are encouraged to remain on NRT as those who complete the programme are more likely to stay stopped. Successful group members are now entitled to attend monthly ex-smokers' meetings. Invitations are sent out to all for up to one year. Relapse is common when people become complacent, so members discuss how this might happen and decide on avoidance tactics.

Help for those who relapse

Those who do not manage to stop during the six-week session are asked why they think this happened. Maybe now was not the right time for them and they will need to think about what triggered a return to smoking. Advisers always suggest they try again and not to feel discouraged. They are assured that they will succeed once they identify what is standing in the way. They are advised to contact the support group again in three months' time to discuss beginning a new programme.

An ex-smoker's story

'I surprised myself I gave up but I couldn't have done it on my own. It was the helpful and friendly staff at the local service who gave me the support and encouragement I needed. Thanks Bexley Stop Smoking Service, Jo Woodvine and Jan.' Karen McCabe.

One-to-one support

Some people prefer one-to-one help and support. In many areas, trained advisers offer this help tailored to individual needs. You'll need to make an appointment to arrange it.

⊘ The GP's role

Most GP practices run support groups or advice clinics. GPs refer patients to the practice nurse for ongoing support, once they have decided that they want to quit. However, sometimes the right moment arises in a consultation, for example, regarding a smoking-related medical condition, and triggers a quit attempt. Then the doctor can prescribe nicotine patches to patients and ask them to return, to monitor their progress.

A GP's story

'Helping a patient stop smoking is tremendously rewarding from a GP's point of view. I remember a man in his late fifties who had tried many times to quit. He was suffering from quite severe emphysema. I knew that stopping smoking was the only thing that would help his chronic chest condition. We talked about his smoking. He told me his wife complained that she had to keep washing the curtains. I prescribed nicotine patches and asked him to come back to see me again. When he returned, I was amazed to see that his complexion had changed from grey to a healthy pink. He had stopped smoking after our talk and he (and his wife) were so delighted. He managed to stay off cigarettes. Smoking is so damaging to every system in the body, and to those who do not choose to smoke. It is distressing to see small children brought in with chest and ear infections caused by passive smoke exposure in the home. Thankfully, we can help with advice, support, prescriptions and referral to NHS services. More and more smokers are finding the way out of this life-threatening addiction.' Dr Dawn Milner, Shropshire

❯ The pharmacist's role

All community pharmacists have been engaged in helping people to stop smoking since NRT became available over the counter in 1991. They offer advice and support for smokers, helping customers choose the most suitable type of NRT product for them and ensuring they use the right dose.

A pharmacist's story

'My experience is that those attempting to quit rarely need explanations about the damage smoking causes. Even young children know that smoking kills. No sane person wants their child to start smoking, to be exposed to second-hand smoke or be denied a smoke-free environment. Some smokers worry that they can overdose using patches or will experience unwelcome side effects such as rashes and nightmares and won't be able to shower or swim. I remove these misconceptions and explain the overwhelming benefits of using NRT. It could be argued that successful quitters are mentally prepared to be at the end of their smoking careers by the time they turn up at the pharmacy and seek professional help. This is not the case as I see hundreds of people a year who I help decide to stop and am then able to support them to successfully quit.' Andrew McCoig, Croydon

⊗ Help for pregnant women

Special services are available for women who are pregnant, or trying to start a family, or have babies under one year old. Doncaster's Stop Smoking Service for pregnant women was named one of the best in the country by the Department of Health. The service offers friendly, non-judgemental, tailored support and is run by two specially trained midwives.

Behind the scenes at a service for pregnant women

Lisa Fendall one of the service providers at Doncaster's Stop Smoking Service explained what they do:

'We feel being midwives puts us in the best position to deliver smoking cessation to pregnant women. Our clients sometimes experience pregnancy-related problems and because we are midwives, we can assess and act accordingly. We often liaise with the maternity unit and our professional colleagues to arrange hospital admission or further assessment. There are many factors that

influence the smoking behaviour of pregnant women.
We understand how difficult it is to give up smoking,
especially when other people in the home continue
to smoke. To address this issue we offer advice to the
whole family. We have noticed that quit attempts made
together increase the likelihood of everyone's success. The
health of other children in the house improves when they
are no longer exposed to second-hand smoke. Helping
pregnant women stop smoking is not an easy task but
we have found our friendly flexible service has been very
successful.'

To encourage women to use the service they allow clients to decide where and when the most convenient time and place is to meet. They can offer one-to-one appointments in the client's home or at another venue of their choice. This can be their workplace, GP's surgery or the antenatal clinic to coincide with a scan or hospital appointment. Working patterns are considered and some evening appointments can be given.

An ex-smoker's story

'The last time I tried to give up I felt frustrated because
my partner smoked around me. I wasn't able to manage
it. The help and support on offer through the NHS is
much better now. I've been seen by an adviser who is
also a qualified midwife. She understands about smoking
and the risks to the baby. This is really helpful as I'm
trying to get pregnant again. She has explained all about
fertility and given me some great tips but I know stopping
smoking is the number one thing I have to do. I'm now on
NRT and feel confident that with the help available, I will
be successful.' Deborah Tuite.

⟩ Stop-smoking courses in the workplace

Many employers offer in-house courses to help staff stop smoking. By allowing time off to attend group sessions and providing free treatment products they make this an attractive option for employees. It is a great investment from a company perspective, too, as staff health and absenteeism will improve. A typical programme might run for around an hour and a half each week for eight weeks and covers:

○ Smoking and addiction.

○ Stress reduction.

○ Increasing self-esteem.

○ Relaxation techniques.

○ Personal investment.

○ Implementing positive lifestyle changes.

> Behind the scenes at a workplace stop-smoking programme
>
> Caroline Douglas manages the UCLH Trust Stop Smoking Service and runs a staff stop smoking support programme. She explains:
>
> *'Many report they expected to find stopping very difficult and unpleasant, and instead find they are enjoying not smoking because of the programme. The trust has found that it helps staff successfully stop smoking if they take the trouble to attend the group regularly, and learn to invest in themselves and make positive lifestyle changes.'*

A workplace support programme

The following NHS programme is typical:

Week one

Staff are assessed for suitability, based on their motivation and commitment to stopping smoking. If it's the right time, they are provided with NRT and coaching to help them quit. Their carbon monoxide levels are measured weekly.

Week two

The second week focuses on stress and how to respond in a positive way. Staff are taught techniques to relax and calm their mind and to help them manage stress. They are often surprised to find that they are not experiencing the mood swings and severe withdrawal symptoms they feared when the use NRT.

Weeks two to eight

Progress is monitored on a weekly basis and at the end of the eight-week programme those who have successfully quit smoking get a certificate to mark their achievement.

⊘ Services for ethnic communities

There are specialised smoking cessation services aimed at ethnic communities as well. They often provide targeted help aimed at those giving up tobacco products other than cigarettes. One example is a tobacco cessation service set up in Slough, Berkshire, to address the high smoking rates in the town. Over 10,000 people in Slough suffer from high blood pressure. The majority are from the Asian community and the condition is often a direct result of smoking. Tobacco use in this population includes chewing tobacco and the water pipe (hookah or shisha).

Chewing tobacco is popular among the South Asian community and is considered a part of tradition, particularly among women. There are strong barriers against giving up, especially as products such as Zarda and Gutka are readily available in local shops and cost as little as 20p.

Water pipes use a hot coal atop a wad of flavoured tobacco; the smoke is bubbled through the water, and the smoker then inhales. There are new locations opening up across the UK, where visitors can sit down and smoke these pipes.

Behind the scenes at a smoking cessation service for ethnic groups

Leena Sankla, project director of Cardio Wellness, which set-up the Slough smoking cessation service explains more about her work:

'We set up easily accessible clinics in convenient and safe locations to meet the needs of the ethnic population. Many users are unaware of the health risks of chewing tobacco and the high levels of nicotine that some of these products contain. In some people their addiction level is so high they use these products throughout the night. Use of water pipes, such as the Arabian hookah is growing in popularity among young Asian people. Hookah use is also very popular amongst Asian women where shisha parties are held as a means of social interaction. The work we are doing is essential as there is a higher prevalence of tobacco-related illness within the ethnic community, such as heart disease and oral cancer. We deliver help on a confidential one-to-one basis in a number of different languages including Hindu, Urdu, Punjabi, Gujarati – and now Polish.' www.cardio-wellness.com

⊗ QUIT®

QUIT is an independent charity that helps smokers to stop and has already helped over two million smokers. The Quitline®, 0800 00 22 00, is open until 9 p.m., seven days a week, and is run by a trained counselling team. The QUIT team offers free and confidential telephone counselling for any smoker preparing to quit, or wanting to talk about difficulties they're experiencing while quitting, including withdrawal symptoms, cravings and peer and family pressure. The team also offers support to the family and friends of smokers, and to teachers worried about their pupils smoking. The team can refer callers to the different departments of QUIT if necessary.

QUIT email service

Smokers who prefer to email from their desk at work, or at home in the evenings, can send a message to stopsmoking@ quit.org.uk for personalised same-day advice. Many quitters find it helpful to re-read personal replies whenever they need help staying focused.

Asian Quitline®
www.asianquitline.org

The bilingual counselling team runs five Asian helplines: in Bengali, Urdu, Punjabi, Gujarati and Hindi. They offer confidential and sensitive advice and free informative leaflets in these languages. The service, supported by the British Heart Foundation, helps Asian smokers discuss the cultural issues surrounding smoking, and stops language being a barrier. Even those Asian smokers who speak English fluently use the service because they can discuss the cultural issues surrounding smoking with someone who understands. Both male and female, young and old appreciate this special service for the Asian community.

Young people

Young people calling Quitline, or emailing the counsellors, can ask for special resources designed with them in mind, including postcards and stickers, and discuss issues personal to them, such as peer pressure or concerns about family members who smoke. Teachers worried about smoking among pupils can be referred to the Youth Services Development team. The team runs a youth programme 'Break Free', which visits schools, youth clubs and attends community events across the UK. The aim is to help the young make informed choices about smoking – in a lively and interactive way.

❯ Top tips

- NHS Smoking Helpline is a source of practical, non-judgemental advice and support on giving up smoking.
- The Helpline gives details of local NHS Stop Smoking Services and offers free information packs.
- NHS Pregnancy Smoking Helpline 0800 169 9 169 is for women who want to stop smoking during pregnancy.
- The NHS Asian Tobacco Helpline offers specific advice for ethnic communities.
- Local smoking cessation groups provide advice, support and encouragement to those who want to quit in a group setting.
- One-to-one advice is also available.
- Many companies offer workplace programmes to help staff quit smoking.
- Quitline – 0800 00 22 00 – is run by the independent charity QUIT and offers support to smokers and their family and friends.
- QUIT also runs specialist services for Asian smokers, young people and teachers worried about pupils who smoke.

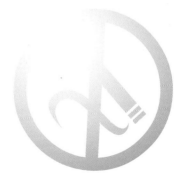

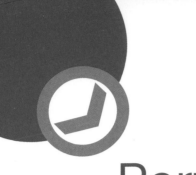

Part 2
TIME
TO
QUIT

'Today is the beginning of your smoke-free life...'

Chapter 6
Quit Day!

The big day is coming! Your quit date is on the horizon and soon you'll stop smoking for good. It may seem daunting, but don't fret – remember, many others have been there before you, and if they managed to do it so can you!

Sometimes a hurdle seems big because you spend so much time worrying about it, rather than planning a way to tackle it. Giving up smoking is not one big challenge but rather a series of small ones, none of which is too big to manage. In this section I'll help you to separate them all out and see what they're really made of. Everyone who really *wants* to stop smoking *can* stop smoking, and there is plenty of help available.

An ex-smoker's story

'Where I work, a lot of people still smoke and, even though it sounds silly, at break times I choose to sit in the smoke room with my friends. Instead of having a cigarette I drink fruit juice. If I feel tempted to smoke, I say to myself "Which would you rather do – smoke a cigarette or look at a picture of your child smiling at you?" Then I take out my mobile phone and look through the pictures of my family and son.' Michael Logan

---

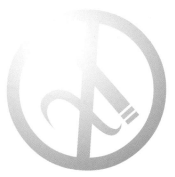

❯ Break your smoking routines

People who plan how they are going to cope once they give up are more likely to succeed than those who don't. Start by emptying your house, car and so on of cigarettes, lighters, matches and other materials related to smoking to clear away temptation in readiness for the day you are going to quit. Now think about all your old smoking habits, as planning ways to manage these beforehand will put you ahead of the game.

Most smokers find that smoking is linked with a particular routine, such as a regular activity or method of behaviour. Changing routines can go a long way towards breaking the habit of lighting up at certain times of the day. Now work out a coping strategy for dealing with all the times or situations that might tempt you back into smoking. For example, if you have a cigarette when you first wake up, to prepare you for the day, you could have a shower instead. Then eat a proper breakfast. A fresh fruit juice will help to wake you up. A good tip is to keep strong mouthwash in the fridge. After eating a meal, rinse out your mouth, as this makes you less likely to have cigarette after eating. Don't linger at the dinner table but get up and do something, such as the washing up.

❯ Dealing with temptation

There will be times when it will seem more difficult to resist temptation. At these moments it may seem easier just to light up and forget all about wanting to stop smoking. You need to understand this feeling and expect it to happen. As you go through the process of quitting, avoid temptation by becoming aware of trigger situations. Be on your guard at mealtimes, when drinking alcohol, working under pressure, family occasions and when out celebrating.

List your personal triggers to smoke

Think about your personal triggers and what you will do to resist them and take the time to fill in the answers in the charts below.

Smoking triggers

☐   Seeing someone else light up

☐

☐

☐

☐

☐

☐

☐

☐

Alternative activities instead of smoking

☐   Go for a walk

☐

☐

☐

☐

☐

☐

☐

☐

❯ Adjusting to change

All change requires time and effort to adjust. When you stop smoking, it's natural to wonder if you are doing the right thing and whether or not it is really worth it. If you recall the number of years you have been smoking, it's easy to see why it may take a while to come to terms with changing such a long-established habit. Even if you don't feel 100 per cent sure, you need to find a way to push away any doubts and carry on.

Ask yourself, 'If I don't stop, what could happen to me?'
Write the answer here.

Tips to change the way you think about smoking:

Don't get caught up in a tug of war between wanting to stop and wanting to smoke. The following tips will help you let go of negative thoughts and change the way you think about smoking:

- Recognise that 'just one' cigarette can undo all your hard work.
- Remember that *you* are in control of what you do – not the cigarettes.
- Remind yourself of why *you* want to stop and the benefits you will get.
- Remember that *you* are *choosing* not to smoke. No one can make you.
- Take it one day at a time – don't worry about tomorrow or next week.

Tips to help you cope with the urge to smoke:

- Remember that each craving to smoke will pass in a few minutes.
- Sit still and take three long slow deep breaths.
- Drink a glass of water very slowly.
- Call someone up and talk about what's going on and how you feel.
- Check if you are using enough of your treatment product

Tips to help you lighten or change your mood:

- Say to yourself, 'I intend to be smoke free.'
- Take each hour as it comes, remember that even 'bad' times don't last forever.
- Remind yourself that you are in charge of all the choices you make.
- You are not losing a friend, you are regaining control of your life.
- Be reassured that each negative feeling or thought that you experience, however difficult it may seem at the time, will pass eventually.

❯ Handling social situations

Many smokers find it much easier if they make a general announcement to their social circle about stopping smoking. By doing this everyone knows what they are up to and can be prepared for the changes ahead. Telling friends and family about quitting can open up new avenues of support and encouragement. There is no right way to handle this. Some people decide to stop in secret so they can enjoy surprising their family when they announce the news. Think about what would work best for you among your social circle. Have you told people about your plans? If not, why not? List your reasons below.

Reasons for not telling others that you plan to stop:

☐

☐

☐

An ex-smoker's story

'They say that in order to stop, you have to find your own personal key reason. Of course I knew about the health reasons, but maybe staying alive wasn't the most important thing to me. Money was a strong issue as I do like to save my money, but that was not a strong enough motivation to stop. I heard someone say that when we buy cigarettes we are being conned by tobacco companies, and though that also struck a fairly strong chord with me, still it was not my "key". What finally did it for me was vanity. I read that chemicals in cigarettes are stored in fat cells that become cellulite. I didn't need any contributions to that part of my body! So that was what made me stop. I am amazed at how strong the craving is sometimes even to this day. I have the odd one from a friend, maybe once a year. It goes straight to my head and tastes foul so I never even finish it, but

*still the thought is there and about 10 or 12 months
later I have another one, when particularly stressed.'*
Cindy Sykes

Maybe you've got friends who wouldn't be too supportive of what
you're doing. Ask yourself, is now the best time to meet up with
them or should I delay it? Other smokers may feel threatened
by your attempts to stop. They may have tried in the past and
been unsuccessful. Your success may somehow make them feel
bad and they may keep bugging you to light up. You will need to
deal with them firmly. Despite what anyone says, you know the
benefits of what you are doing.

What will you say to other smokers?

☐   **No thanks I don't smoke**

☐

☐

Avoid getting into arguments about it. Everyone seems to
know an elderly person who still smokes 40 a day and remains
fit and healthy. If you are feeling vulnerable, these arguments
may tip the balance in the favour of you going back to smoking.
For every long-living, chain-smoking grandmother your friends
talk about, there are thousands of smokers who die before their
time as a result of their addiction to nicotine.

The truth is, smoking is a gamble. One out of every two
lifelong smokers dies as a result of their smoking. Never let
another person's opinions get through to you – because no
one who smokes knows how the odds are stacked. Like all
current topics of conversation, the good news is, after a while
your smoke-free status won't even be up for discussion. You
never know, your would-be saboteurs may eventually follow your
example.

An ex-smoker's story

'I'd always been happy smoking. One or two of my friends had quit but I couldn't see the point as most of my family smoked. Then I met a really nice guy who didn't smoke, and after a couple of years we decided we wanted to get married. I knew he would prefer it if I didn't smoke but he never nagged me. Four months before our wedding date I got sick with one of my frequent colds and I was given antibiotics. They made me feel so ill I didn't fancy a cigarette. While I was lying in bed I decided what a lovely wedding present it would be for my husband if I stopped smoking. As I got better I was tempted to relapse. But then I found the most beautiful wedding dress. It was perfect but too expensive. I sat down and worked out how much I could save by not smoking and found I would actually be able to afford it. My decision to stop smoking helped me to look like a princess on my wedding day and my husband was thrilled with his new non-smoking bride.'
Siobhan D.

❯ Change the way you think about smoking

While breaking the physical addiction to nicotine is hard, for many smokers breaking the habit – the psychological addiction – is harder. This is mainly because smoking has become deeply ingrained over the years and so has become an integral part of your life. Happy or sad, bored or when concentrating, relaxed or stressed, cigarettes played a part in almost all situations, so tell yourself the following:

Reminders of why you want to stop
- I want to have a smoke-free lifestyle.
- I want the benefits.
- I want to live longer.
- No one is making me change.
- I have decided to stop smoking – this is my own free choice.

Don't feel resentful. Even if there are times when you wonder why you are doing this to yourself, remember that you'll soon be free from the grip of nicotine addiction and these negative thoughts will stop.

Are you ready to stop smoking for good?

My main reason for stopping smoking is...

How do I expect to feel when I've succeeded?

Is there something I might miss about smoking?

Is there something I might lose because I no longer smoke?

Are there any relationships that may change when I've stopped smoking?

What will I gain from going back to smoking?

Having completed this exercise, can you spot any dangerous assumptions or ideas you need to pay attention to? If so, ask yourself if thinking in this way could set you up for relapse. Talk to your supportive friends or call the NHS Smoking Helpline. An adviser can help you explore your thinking and emotional attachment to smoking.

An ex-smoker's story

'I tried many times to give up but when anything went wrong in my life, I reached for the packet. Eventually, I knew I had got to the point where if my future was to be successful, my attempt to quit had to be successful too. I decided to go on an unusual holiday to start my cigarette-free life. I chose to visit the gorillas in Rwanda – you can't buy cigarettes in the mountains of Africa. The holiday was one I shall never forget – one of my greatest memories. I felt wonderful on my return, healthy, rested, fit and determined never to let myself down by smoking again.'
Lynn Williamson

❯ Final preparations

It's always a good idea to make some last minute checks to be sure you have everything ready for the first day of your smoke-free lifestyle.

Before the quit date

○ Old habits can take time to change so practise the new ones.

○ Look at your list of reasons for stopping smoking and copy them onto a card to carry around with you. If you have a moment of temptation, read your list to help you refocus on your goal.

○ Join a NHS Stop Smoking Service support group. The NHS Smokers Helpline (0800 169 0 169) can give you the contact details for your local stop smoking support services.

- Visit your general practitioner, practice nurse or pharmacist to ask about the products suitable for you that will help you manage the nicotine withdrawal symptoms.
- Use nicotine treatment products, such as NRT or Zyban, if you feel you need them.
- Look over your ideas for managing the first few days without cigarettes and practise some of the changes before the quit date.
- If you get stuck thinking of alternative things to do instead of smoking, decide if you need to spend a bit longer preparing yourself. Working around a date for which you are not ready may set you up to relapse.
- Decide what you are going to say to yourself if you get tempted to smoke.
- Plan a new activity to keep your hands and mind occupied.

An ex-smoker's story

'I treated myself to personal coaching and was taught to do relaxation, which really helped. This in turn helped me cope with the stress of not smoking and the cravings too. Being part of a group was fantastic as it meant meeting up each week and getting support from others who were feeling the same way as me. My work magazine was interested in featuring a story about me quitting and what experiences I was having. This meant all my work colleagues knew I was giving up and they were able to encourage and support me too. This really gave me the incentive to continue my quit attempt. I now encourage other friends who smoke to keep trying and not give in. Since quitting I've really felt great, have more money and everything smells sweeter.' Gill Tew

❯ Managing the First 24 Hours

The following suggestions are designed to help you get through your first smoke-free day.

- Talk to a friend/relative about your plans and why stopping is important for you. Ask them to give you support.
- Team up with someone else who is quitting – a 'support buddy' – and help each other.
- Talk to an ex-smoker. Find out how they stopped – and believe that you can too.
- Call the NHS Smoking Helpline on 0800 169 0 169.
- Say 'no' to any jobs that put you under too much pressure.
- Wash your hair – you'll feel fresh all day and not be reminded of the smell of cigarettes.
- Treat yourself to some nice-smelling candles or flowers for your home.
- Wash or dry clean your clothes before you stop. That way everything will smell fresher, and help keep you motivated.
- Remember to laugh and smile! You're going to be free from addiction!
- Keep your list of motivations to stop smoking close at hand, to help you achieve your goal. Perhaps stick them on the fridge at home, and on your computer or around your working area when at work.
- Socialise with people who do not smoke.
- Plan your social activities around smoke-free places.
- Sitting around may cause temptation, so keep active.
- Go out in the fresh air and if possible take a walk.
- Think about what's worked for you in the past – and what hasn't – and make use of your experiences.
- Put the money you save in a jar and watch it mount up.
- Keep a calendar or wall chart and mark every day you've been smoke-free (see page 112).

Smoke-free day wall chart

Tick off each smoke-free day on the chart below and write the reward you have given yourself in the box at the end of the row.

				Monday
				Tuesday
				Wednesday
				Thursday
				Friday
				Saturday
				Sunday
				Reward

❯ Managing the First Week

During the first week you'll be aware of your decision to stop smoking on almost an hour-by-hour basis. You may also have to battle against any 'little' ideas that pop into your head about 'how nice smoking again might be' and how 'just one couldn't hurt'. This takes willpower. It is really important to recognise that one cigarette feeds the nicotine addiction and within a few hours you will be back in the same place – except this time you will be smoking. You have set a goal to stop smoking. You can do it. The days ahead will get easier but if you give in at this stage you will have to go right back to the beginning and start again.

I will respond to the urge to smoke by telling myself

Managing the early days

As a non-smoker you need to change the way you think, the way you talk and even the way you act. Take each hour at a time and give yourself frequent rests and breaks. If you're finding some moments tough, look back over the list of reasons you want to stop smoking. Even if it seems hard at first, a big part of you believes it will be worth all the effort! Trust that part of you and be patient with yourself.

Try these distraction techniques
- Take a few slow, deep breaths if you feel stressed.
- Drink a glass of water slowly.
- Go for a quick stroll in the fresh air if possible.
- Busy your thoughts by doing a logic puzzle, Sudoku or crossword.
- Chat to a friend who makes you laugh.

If you are faced with a problem
- Be honest with yourself – ask, 'What is the real issue?'
- Think about what you could differently, then try doing it!
- Talk problems over with someone you trust.

Use time management
- Sort out what you have to do.
- Plan your time so you do the most important tasks first.
- Make realistic plans for achieving your short- and long-term goals.
- Take each hour and day as it comes.

Put yourself first
- Every day, do one thing that's just for you.
- Practise saying 'no' – and don't feel guilty about it.
- Make sure you go to bed on time and try to get enough sleep.
- Do something that interests you, or find a new hobby.

Relax

O Take some time out for yourself – even 15 minutes will help.

O Sit somewhere quiet, turn off your phone and relax.

O Go swimming or walking, or join a new activity group.

O Listen to some music you enjoy, or read a good book.

Keep your spirits up

O Watch the money you used to spend on cigarettes mount up.

O Continue to mark off each smoke-free day on your calendar (see page 112).

O Watch a comedy. Laughing always helps you feel better.

O Congratulate yourself every day on being successful.

> An ex-smoker's story
>
> *'Change your whole way of thinking towards smoking. On previous attempts I always felt that I was missing out on something. Now I look upon it as something that used to be a part of my life but is no longer and that I am not being deprived of anything.'* Lynda Munns

❯ Refusing cigarettes

It's not easy to refuse a cigarette, especially if you've never done it before. Learning to say 'no' is an important part of good communication. If you are worried about friends taking offence when you refuse their offer of a cigarette, why not start off all conversations by reminding them you have stopped smoking. If a new acquaintance offers you a cigarette, simply reply, 'No thanks, I don't smoke.'

Don't say, 'I'm trying to stop.' Many smokers find that telling people they are *trying* to give up leaves them wide open to further remarks like:

- 'Just one more won't make any difference.'
- 'Any damage is already done, so go on – enjoy yourself!'
- 'I can't see what all the fuss is about – smoking has never done me any harm.'

Try to avoid getting into these conversations. No explanation and no justification is needed from you. It's your decision to make and you need to stick to it so you can achieve your goal.

Think up some responses you can give if offered a cigarette

One thing to be aware of is that some smokers may feel resentful, annoyed or even jealous when they see someone trying to stop smoking. On the flip side after you have given up, you could feel a bit jealous because they can still smoke. These are all normal feelings and will pass.

Who might try to put hurdles in your way? List their names below:

Make a real effort to avoid the company of these people in your first few weeks. If it's not possible, prepare yourself by being really focused about why you are stopping smoking.

⟩ Ask your family and friends to help

It will help if you can involve your family and friends in your decision to stop smoking. If you live with someone who smokes, it will be much easier to give up together. If your workplace has brought in a smoke-free policy, try to get any colleagues who smoke to join you in quitting. Other people can help you stop smoking by:

Giving lots of verbal support and encouragement

It's taken a lot of courage for you to make the decision – ask them to congratulate you often. Don't let anyone nag or lecture you on the dangers of smoking. It's far better if people are impressed by your effort.

Understanding what you're going through

It's possible you may get moody in the first few weeks. Friends need to realise this is a normal part of the process of giving up. Explain about the physical and emotional effects of stopping smoking so they can be more supportive.

Asking you how you're feeling

You may need to talk about why it's important for you to stop and when you feel tempted to relapse. Ask them to be patient with you if you get irritable. Just let them know this is only a short phase and you will soon be back to normal.

Being there, whatever happens

Remind them that this isn't the time to burden you with their problems. Promise that when you're through the challenge of stopping, you'll be fully there for them too. Ask if they can help with any chores during the first week when you give up – it'll really make a difference to your stress levels.

Encouraging you to carry on

Discuss what situations might lead you to lapsing and having a cigarette and ask for their help in tackling these problems. Even if they are smokers themselves, remind them that they mustn't offer you one, even if you beg. Nor must they be hard on you if you slip up in the early days.

Rewarding you

Why not use the money you've saved to take the family out for a treat. Plan lots of things you can all do together. You'll be less tempted to smoke when you are in a cinema or gym, or playing in the park, than in your local pub.

Remember that it takes time

Some smokers need several attempts before they stop for good. So the support people offer needs to be ongoing and they need to be patient with you.

Involve your children in the quit attempt

Maybe your children can be the ones to record your progress by ticking the chart. You could also use some of the money you save to take them on a family outing. If they are involved with your goal, they are more likely to understand if you get in a bad mood or act irritable. Ask them to give you a hug if they spot these signs. Let them know what you are going through. Remind them how important it is that they never start smoking because they would only end up facing the same challenge.

> **An ex-smoker's story**
>
> *'I stopped smoking when my 12-year-old daughter started crying because she was frightened that I wouldn't be around to see her grow up. This gave me the impetus I needed to stop. I told everyone I knew and most people went out of their way to encourage me. Most helpful were my family and work colleagues who knew how many failed*

attempts I'd had in the past. Stopping smoking is worth it as I have more money, I'm able to taste food and my clothes don't stink like an old ashtray!' Neil Thompson

Managing the second week

You've done an amazing job to go seven days without smoking. Don't underestimate this. Review your progress and you'll soon see how far you've come. Each and every day you have been breaking an old habit and practising new ones – well done for keeping going. You've also been learning what support you need, who's there when you want to talk and importantly, how to cope with the withdrawal symptoms.

You've started the journey, you've turned the first corner, but there's still some climbing to do. You are changing from someone who has been a smoker to someone who is free from smoke. You had to *learn* to smoke. Now you have to *learn* to stop.

An ex-smokers' story

'Understand that it is a "Want" and a "Desire" to smoke – not a NEED. It all comes down to you and whether you choose to smoke or not.' Neil Butlin

Learning to be a non-smoker

When you think about it, the title 'smoker' is quite judgemental. No one is born a smoker. It's a habit a person has to learn. Do you remember trying your first cigarette? You may recall coughing, choking, feeling dizzy or even sick. As smoking is difficult to master at first it probably took you a while to get into the habit. Stopping smoking will take practice, too. What you are doing is letting go of old habits, which when you think about it, were not really part of your identity before that first cigarette. You are not giving up something – you are going back to something you always were – a person who doesn't smoke. You have made the choice to be free and ultimately even if it's tough going for the next few weeks, this decision will make your life easier.

By now you will have experienced some of the effects of nicotine withdrawal. How have you been getting on? How have you been feeling? Don't put yourself through a difficult period of 'cold turkey', if you haven't done so already check out the wide range of NRT products available to help you manage the symptoms.

An ex-smoker's story

'I smoked on–off, on–off for years. In the end it was for money and love that I quit. Having a partner who didn't like me smoking helped the most – he both motivated my quit attempt and supported me. It was worth it! I got his kisses in exchange for disgusting fags! Non-smokers encouraging smokers to quit are a powerful force! He died last year and I will forever owe him for keeping me to be smoke–free.' Cecilia Farren

❯ Top tips

- Plan ahead to help you cope with stressful situations.
- Before you stop, remove as many temptations as possible – get rid of all reminders of smoking such as ashtrays and lighters, throw away any cigarettes on or near you and don't buy any more.
- Pair up with a 'support buddy' and help each other.
- Contact your local NHS Stop Smoking Service for practical help and advice from trained specialists.
- Use nicotine replacement therapy or Zyban to help you manage the cravings.
- Avoid situations and people that might tempt you to smoke.
- Keep back some of the money you're saving – and treat yourself!
- Promise yourself that you will never ask a smoker for a cigarette.

- There's no such thing as having 'just one' cigarette. Don't do it!
- Take it one day at a time and congratulate yourself every day.
- Think positive: tell yourself you CAN do it!

Chapter 7
Managing Challenges

Life isn't always easy or fair. Just as you are feeling on top of your quit attempt it's possible something could happen that makes you think returning to smoking is a good idea. You always have a free choice. Don't let this event become an excuse to light up. Ask yourself, 'Will smoking help me face this in the long run?'

It's important to try to recognise those things you cannot change. Look closely at the problem. If there's no hope of achieving the outcome you want, why not let the issue go and deal with the next step rather than getting worked up and relapsing in the process.

⊘ How to handle the desire to smoke

If you are having a really bad time, it can help to talk to someone about what you are going through. The NHS Helpline is open from 7 a.m. to 11 p.m. Call and talk to an adviser about your problem. Here are some more tips and suggestions. Tick the ones that appeal and add your own solutions to the list.

Instant substitutes for craving:
- Put an NRT aid in your mouth such as nicotine gum, nicotine micro tab or nicotine lozenge to boost your nicotine level and reduce your desire to smoke.
- Cut a straw into cigarette-sized pieces and inhale fresh air through the straw.
- During stressful moments, take a few long, slow, deep breaths.
- Sip a glass of iced water or diluted fruit juice slowly.

- Keep your hands occupied – play with a stress ball, worry beads or a pen or pencil.
- Call the NHS Smoking Helpline on 0800 169 0 169.
- Do some light exercise or go for a short walk.
- Avoid too much coffee, tea or alcohol.
- Buy sugar-free sweets and gum.
- Suck a glucose tablet – they trigger the release of 'feel-good' chemicals in the brain.
- After eating, brush your teeth and rinse out with a strong mouthwash. Notice how much cleaner your breath is now you've given up.
- Tell yourself, 'I choose to stop smoking.'
- Keep a notebook and pen near the phone and doodle while chatting.
- Play your favourite music and sing along to the tracks.
- Invite someone to join you and cook a meal for them.

If you've got more time:
- Have a relaxing shower or a bath.
- Count up how much money you've saved since giving up.
- Do a job on your 'to do' list.
- Rekindle an old friendship. Call or contact an old friend.
- Prepare yourself something special to eat and savour every mouthful.

Long-term distractions:
- Take up a hobby that keeps your hands busy, such as painting, knitting, learning a musical instrument or hobby crafting.
- Decorate your home to get rid of any tobacco smells.
- Take up a new sport or active hobby.

Get out and about

Try to identify the cause of the problem and look to see if there is another way to handle it without smoking. Maybe it's possible to change your environment or at least the room you're in. Ideally, go for a walk outside in the fresh air. If that's not easy, just doing something active can really help. How about walking up and down a flight of stairs or a corridor?

Interact with other people

Helping someone else can really make you feel good about yourself. Think about the people you know – is there a non-smoker you can help out? Perhaps an elderly neighbour or a busy friend would appreciate a helping hand? Doing something completely different is a good way to take your mind off smoking, especially if in the process you've made someone else's day better.

Handling worry and stress

New stress management skills can take time to develop. Don't expect to be able to change everything at once and get it 'right' first time. Expecting too much of yourself will only add more stress as you settle into your new non-smoking lifestyle.

Your old habits have taken time to build up and it will take a while to feel comfortable with new ones. It's important not to let the changes associated with stopping smoking stress you out. Watch out for these symptoms and do something about them before they build up or get out of your control.

Signs of mental stress:
- **Worrying about little things.**
- **Finding it hard to concentrate.**
- **Constantly feeling anxious.**
- **Feeling pessimistic.**
- **Being indecisive.**
- **Finding little things more difficult than they should be.**

Signs of physical stress:

- Feeling shaky.
- Having a rapid heartbeat.
- Restlessness.
- Headaches.
- Stomach cramps.
- Diarrhoea.

Many people believe that smoking relieves anxiety or stress. The reality is that most smokers tend to be more stressed than non-smokers. Think of a smoker and a non-smoker caught in a long meeting. Who is more likely to be distracted, fidgety and longing to get out of the meeting room? Whose stress level is likely to be higher in this situation, a smoker's or a nonsmoker's?

When you stop smoking, you are removing an enormous cause of stress from your life and there is no evidence that nicotine enhances a person's performance over non-smokers. If you do feel stressed, how about trying some relaxation exercises, making use of aromatherapy oils, having a warm bath or burning off your frustrations at the gym?

⟩ Make some 'me' time

- Take some time out for yourself each day.
- Set limits for yourself. Practise saying 'no' to difficult jobs if you feel stressed.
- Talk to someone unbiased if you're finding things difficult to manage (including the NHS Smoking Helpline on 0800 169 0 169).
- Go to bed on time and try to get the full amount of sleep you need.
- Sit down and take a few long, slow, deep breaths.
- Do a series of stretches or light exercise.
- Go for a swim or join a keep-fit class/activity group.
- Join a yoga or meditation class.

Let meditation become part of your stress-reduction plan

Just stopping what you're doing and taking some quiet time out of your normal routine to let your mind be still is really beneficial. If you can let this become part of your daily life, the minutes you put aside, particularly in the first few weeks of stopping smoking, will really give you a space that is yours where you can let go of everything that is around you.

Try this relaxation technique

- Wear comfortable clothing.
- Sit or lay down in a comfortable warm spot.
- Close your eyes and imagine a beautiful scene or a place where you've been really happy; maybe a holiday resort or the countryside.
- Keep your eyes closed. Take three slow, very deep breaths. Make sure you fill your lungs completely and let the air out very slowly.
- Starting with your feet, tense and relax your foot muscles by pointing your toes downwards, then letting go.
- Follow this sequence for all your muscles.
- Move your attention slowly up your body, tensing and relaxing your legs, then your abdomen, arms, shoulders and finally your neck and face muscles.
- Finally make your whole body tense, squeezing every muscle, and then let go as you breathe out.
- Repeat this process three times.
- Finally, stay completely still for 10 minutes.

It is worth persisting with this exercise. It may seem a bit strange at first, but you'll soon start to recognise the benefits. Just the physical act of stopping and taking slow, deep breaths can calm you down. And there is a lot of medical evidence that relaxation has many other benefits. Some people say it boosts their self-esteem, concentration and productivity. Try it and see what it can do for you. If you get interested in this type of relaxation, your local library can give you information on meditation groups.

An ex-smoker's story
'Never worry about stopping or mope over what you've lost. Enjoy what you have gained and enjoy the challenge! From the moment you stop – grab life by the horns and enjoy the ride. Share your experiences with others as it really helps!' Matt Hopwood

⊗ New ways to manage your stress

Time management
- Prioritise your daily goals and tasks.
- Schedule your time according to these priorities.
- Set up realistic short- and long-term plans.

Problem solving
- If you feel stuck – ask yourself:
- Exactly what is the core problem?
- What could I do differently?
- DO IT!
- Reflect on the outcome. What changes did this bring about?
- Tell someone else what is going on.

Present moment thinking
- Take stock of all the things that are going well right now.
- Ask yourself, 'What is happening at this exact moment to upset me?'
- Don't let your mind dwell on potential problems or negative outcomes.
- Imagine a perfect ending instead and focus on this for five minutes.

Control your thoughts

- You can control your thoughts by changing your thinking patterns.
- Say to yourself, 'I will be fine, I can do this, I am a successful quitter.'

An ex-smoker's story

'I decided to wash all my clothes, curtains and cushion covers to get rid of the tobacco smell. I rinsed them in a lavender conditioner to make them smell fresh and nice. Then I put pot-pourri and scented candles around the house so everywhere smelt wonderful! Finally I sat back and listened to a relaxation tape with helpful hints on how to relax even further. At the times when I was feeling energetic, I did some knitting, gardening and I even sorted out the greenhouse! I've found it really helpful if I was becoming agitated to go and lie on top of the bed and listen to a relaxing tape.' Christine Hannan

---

Positive affirmations

Positive affirmations can really help you stay focused on your intention to quit. Make sure this is a positive statement, for example, 'It's getting easier everyday,' or 'I *can* do it!' A great tip is to write out one of your goals on a Post-it note and place it in a prominent position. Each time you see it you will be reminded of your focus.

An ex-smoker's story

'Don't let stopping take over your life. If you're thinking constantly about the fact that you're not smoking you are thinking about smoking!' Jo Colls

---

Combating pitfalls

Here are some more common pitfalls that can trap the unwary ex-smoker, so plan what you will do when they appear.

Boredom

This is just a state of mind. Smoking won't change that, but doing something to keep yourself occupied will!

Other smokers

Remind yourself that many smokers wish they didn't have to smoke (just like you used to). They are not enjoying smoking, they're simply feeding an addiction. Real friends won't keep offering you a cigarette. If this gets to be an issue simply take one and break it in half. You'll make your point.

Socialising in the pub

Try to break the connection between drinking and smoking. When you want a drink again, have it at home, away from smokers, and wait until you feel secure enough as a non-smoker before going back to the pub. Try changing your usual drink – it may sound funny, but it really can help break the pattern.

Routines

Certain routines are likely to be inextricably linked with smoking. Many people see smoking as their treat or reward and this association can be hard to break. Break obvious routines. If you always had a cigarette along with a cup of coffee in the morning, try herbal tea or even hot water with lemon (water and cigarette smoke don't taste good together). Or use this time to do something completely different – such as taking the dog for a walk, meditating or going for a swim. Remind yourself that the pleasure you associated with smoking was an illusion. It only seemed good because you were relieving your withdrawal symptoms. This is the basis of all drug addiction.

Tiredness

Feeling tired is normal in the early days of stopping smoking. Exercise is nature's antidote to lethargy and tiredness, and now that you are physically fitter, you'll be surprised at how much easier and more enjoyable exercise can be. Do what works best for you. A regular walk in the park is just as good as an irregular workout in the gym – and your energy levels will soon rise.

Pitfalls chart

The chart on the following page can help you prepare for common pitfalls and either avoid them or cope with them when they arise. In the first column, list any activities you may be involved in that have a strong link to smoking. In the next column, write down the strategies that you have found that have already worked. If you have a possible relapse situation coming up and you haven't worked out how to handle it yet, leave it blank and use the ideas in this chapter to work out a new strategy.

If you get really stuck and there is something coming up you're nervous about, or need a plan, the counsellors at the NHS Smoking Helpline 0800 169 0 169 will be able to assist you in developing a new strategy.

An ex-smoker's story

'I found changing my routine, around the times I would normally smoke, helped me stop. For example, after eating, I used to go to my back door and have a cigarette. Now I spend time playing with my son. I even communicate better with my husband as we have more time to talk about our day. We quite often have a laugh and a joke now.' Dawn Farrell

---

Possible relapse situations	If I get tempted to smoke I will...
Parties, Family Celebrations, Holidays, Meals Out.	*Change plans, Take a buddy, think realistically.*

⟩ Advice if you lapse

A smoker has to learn a new way to run their life by setting up new habits that need to be reinforced. This can take time and a relapse is not uncommon in the first weeks. People who relapse may go through an emotional dip and feel anxious or guilty. If it happens to you, don't judge yourself harshly. Instead, learn from the experience and walk away. It has only been one cigarette and a guilt trip won't do you any good. You need to go back to not smoking and forget it. Most people are receptive to this approach. It may help to share the situation by phoning the NHS Smoking Helpline for emotional support. They can provide lots of ideas or suggestions of new ways to cope.

A setback is simply a sign that that there are still some situations you're not completely comfortable handling yet. Don't be discouraged. Learn from the experience and let it go. Remember to think positively and don't waste time on feeling guilty. Giving up smoking takes practice. It would be a great shame to let a single lapse undo all your hard work and preparation. You didn't fail – you are learning to succeed and sometimes it takes a while to get the hang of stopping smoking.

Each time you stop it helps you understand what works for you, and what would work better next time. Research shows that the more attempts you've had in the past, the more likely you are to succeed in the future. This is because the practical experience and insight you gain each time you relapse gives you a better understanding of the process of stopping. Go back through some of the exercises and charts in this book and work on a new strategy that will help you. The experience you gain from this lapse should make it easier to spot – and deal with – tricky situations in the future.

If you have experienced an early lapse or if you've just had a cigarette DON'T PANIC! Just put it out and start again. Feeling guilty is a waste of time – use your energy for making a fresh start.

To help you get back into a positive frame of mind, think about your reasons for quitting and how good you're going to feel when you've given up. It's a long-term investment and may take a while to adjust to. You have just taken a break on your journey by smoking this cigarette; it doesn't mean you have to go back to the beginning. Be patient with yourself; take it one day at a time. You are learning a new skill called 'Resisting the temptation to smoke'. Very soon you'll be back in full control and rightly proud of your achievement.

Are you really the sort of person who'd let a single lapse undo all your hard work? No I didn't think so! Carry on the good work! You know you can do it!

❯ Getting back on track after a lapse

To help you understand what was going on when you lit up and to make it easier for you to avoid it happening again, answer the questions below. Your answers will help you understand what you have to do to reduce your risk of future relapse.

What were you doing at the time?

Who were you with?

Why did you want a cigarette?

Emotionally, what did it feel like to have that cigarette?

Physically, how did you feel afterwards?

Mentally, how did the experience of smoking compare to your expectation?

Did smoking change the situation or the outcome?

Could you have survived without smoking?

In hindsight, what other options did you have?

What would you do differently another time?

⊘ Top tips

- O Tell everyone you know you do not smoke.
- O Think of yourself as a non smoker.
- O Act like a non-smoker by not smoking.

If you lapse:

- O Make a new decision and stop smoking again immediately.
- O Throw away any remaining cigarettes and do not buy any more.
- O Get away from the place or situation that made you want to smoke.
- O Remind yourself of the reasons you are stopping smoking.
- O Tell yourself why you choose not to smoke.
- O Visualise yourself handling the 'situation' next time without having a cigarette.
- O Call a friend or the NHS Smoking Helpline 0800 169 0 169.

Chapter 8
Managing Symptoms

When you give up smoking you can go through many different physical and emotional processes, which collectively are known as 'withdrawal symptoms'. Not everyone experiences every symptom or to the same extent, but they tend to last between four and twelve weeks. In order to cope with the symptoms you are feeling you may find it helpful to understand exactly what is happening inside your body when you stop using tobacco.

Physical symptoms are likely to start a few hours after you've stopped smoking. They peak within three or four days, then steadily decrease and fade away within three or four weeks. Try to accept that this is simply your body crying out for a drug that it got used to receiving over many years.

⊗ Physical effects

Immediately after quitting, many smokers experience a range of problems such as strong cravings to smoke, light-headedness, changes to your bowel habit, coughing fits, sore gums or mouth. Ex-smokers may feel edgy, hungry, more tired and more short-tempered than usual, and have trouble sleeping. These symptoms are the result of the body clearing itself of nicotine, which is a very powerful addictive chemical.

Nicotine withdrawal may make you restless, irritable, frustrated, tired, sleepless, or accident prone – but these feelings will soon pass. It's important to remember that once you've made it through the early physical withdrawal period, your body will continue its amazing journey of self-repair. The physical addiction to nicotine is fairly brief and all the nicotine will leave your body within 48 hours, once you stop smoking.

From the moment you put out your last cigarette, the body starts to recover. Your body is finding a way to clear out the debris and toxins that have accumulated during your time as a smoker. Although the early stages can cause a certain amount of discomfort, you'll soon feel your body coming back to life. These signs are positive and symptoms will eventually pass after a few weeks. The good news is that things start to get better quite quickly, especially if you use a treatment product to help you wean yourself off nicotine. You will start to notice a big difference in how much better you look and feel.

Even if you have never tried to stop smoking you will be aware of some of the withdrawal and recovery symptoms you can experience. Each time you will have had to go without a cigarette, you will have felt your body's immediate response. These symptoms can all be managed, they are not an excuse to change your mind and go back to smoking.

There are so many places now where you cannot smoke, such as restaurants, cinemas, theatres, public transport, that even committed smokers cannot avoid suffering temporary withdrawal symptoms. But once you make the decision to give up, you know that these symptoms will improve and eventually vanish altogether. Smokers who choose not to give up face suffering these symptoms again and again.

Knowing what to expect when you stop and having a clear idea of how you are going to go through and manage the process of withdrawal and the recovery symptoms is really important. The rest of this chapter explains what is happening to your body in more detail and offers hints and tips to help you cope.

An ex-smoker's story

'The last time I tried to give up I started smoking again because I was feeling particularly low in mood. But I always regretted starting again. I really believe you have to find your own reasons for giving up and a method that suits you as an individual. This time I altered many habits, like not having a cigarette with a cup of tea in the morning, or on my break, which was difficult at first but now I don't even think about it. Whatever the choice in front of me, I know I'd rather not be smoking! My appetite went through the roof at first so I did eat a lot more, particularly chocolate to help me cope. Subsequently I put on around 10 pounds. But my appetite is now more stable and I have learned to resist the temptation of chocolate in the same way that I have had to resist the temptation of a cigarette!' Helena Stephens

What will happen to me?

This table shows the key symptoms, how long they are likely to last and what percentage of quitters are affected by them

Withdrawal effects	Duration	% affected
Light-headedness	up to 48 hours	10
Sleep disturbance	up to 1 week	25
Poor concentration	up to 2 weeks	60
Craving	up to 2 weeks	70
Irritability/aggression	up to 4 weeks	50
Depression	up to 4 weeks	60
Restlessness	up to 4 weeks	60
Increased appetite	up to 10 weeks	70

An ex-smoker's story

'I'd been a smoker for 20 years (on and off) and had tried to stop between 15 and 20 times. My relapses were caused by putting on weight, being tempted whilst under the influence of alcohol, emotional upset, giving

in to a craving. When I first gave up smoking, all I could think about was what I was missing. I obsessed about lighting up and how wonderful it would feel. I didn't give in because my partner was so sure I couldn't do it and I was determined to prove him wrong. After a while, whole days went by when I didn't even think of a cigarette. Now, I laugh at myself for wondering how I could have got into the state I was in! I do not miss smoking at all. In fact, I'm now much freer to plan my time and activities than I ever was being a smoker.' Janet Evans

⊘ How to manage the symptoms

There are many different physical and mental symptoms smokers report experiencing when they give up. It's unlikely that an individual smoker will experience all the symptoms listed. Remember, they are not permanent and they can all be managed.

A good overall tip is to focus on what you are gaining, not what you are 'losing' and give yourself frequent rewards. These don't have to be chocolate or savoury nibbles. Sometimes just sitting down for five minutes and reading, looking out of a window or listening to some music will help. The symptoms of nicotine withdrawal include:

Cravings

Cravings are an intense desire to smoke, which typically lasts only two to three minutes before subsiding. Even when they are violent and catch you unawares, they will still be fleeting. Distracting yourself for the duration of the episode can help. You need to delay the urge as the moment will definitely pass. It helps if you breathe through them by taking deep breaths in and letting out the air gently. Slowly sipping a glass of water will help. The cravings become less frequent and less intense over the first three weeks and should disappear altogether in two to three months. Some people find taking a glucose tablet can help.

Coughing or sore throat

You may have a sore throat and be coughing more than you ever did as a smoker! This is completely normal and temporary. It is a sign that your lungs are doing what they're supposed to do and rejecting the tar and debris that has built up over the years. The millions of tiny hairs (cilia) designed to keep the air passages clean are starting to clear away the dirt caused by cigarette smoke, which can cause a temporary cough. One of the effects of this natural process is that more mucus is produced by your respiratory tract and lungs. A doctor should be consulted if it persists or if you cough up blood.

Constipation

Nicotine is a stimulant and has a laxative effect on which the bowels learn to rely. Constipation is very common in the first week of stopping smoking because your digestive system slows down when nicotine levels are reduced. Providing you drink lots of water and eat plenty of fruit, vegetables and fibre-rich food, your body will quickly get back to normal. If you have also cut down on other stimulants such as tea or coffee, you may be slightly constipated for a bit longer. Don't worry, as your system readjusts it will get back into rhythm and this will pass.

Difficulty concentrating

You may be having difficulty concentrating and in the first few days even some small tasks – like paying bills, for instance – may seem hard. Don't worry, this is normal and it doesn't last. Your brain is simply adjusting to higher levels of oxygen, the loss of carbon monoxide and the absence of nicotine. Try going out for a walk and getting some fresh air and exercise. This is a natural stimulant and within two or three weeks, you will find your concentration levels will begin to get back to normal.

Disturbed sleep/increased dreaming

Disturbed sleep patterns in the early days of stopping smoking are completely normal. Some smokers report night sweats, others that they wake at odd times of the night and can't go back to sleep. It is not uncommon to have an initial week of sleeping badly, followed by a week of difficulty staying awake. These symptoms are unlikely to last longer than a week or two. Try deep breathing and simple relaxation techniques and avoid stimulants, such as coffee, in the hours before you go to bed. A drop of lavender oil on the corner of your pillow can help relax you, or you could try a herbal sleep preparation, available from your pharmacist.

Drug interactions

Stopping smoking may result in slower metabolism and consequent rises in the concentration of some prescription drugs in the blood. For example, the negative effects of smoking on heart rate and blood pressure may mean users of drugs such as beta-blockers need a lower dose when stopping smoking. If you are receiving medical treatment it is important to let your doctor know you are planning to stop in case your treatment regime needs adjustment.

Feeling emotional or having mood swings

You may be feeling very tearful or really irritable. One of the symptoms of nicotine withdrawal is a heightened sense of emotion so you may find yourself either shouting, crying or sulking instead of your normal reaction. Let it out and don't worry that something is wrong with you, this phase passes. This is also totally normal, ask any ex-smoker. These emotional responses can be attributed to the upheaval of breaking a long-established habit and adjusting to the physical problems incurred.

Feelings of loss and grief

Some smokers express strong feelings of 'grief' and loss around the time of giving up smoking. Many say they feel as if they have lost their best friend or even a part of their own identity. These feelings are normal and a grief reaction can occur anytime something is lost from our lives. Grief reactions tend to run in a cycle: denial, anger, bargaining and depression, although not necessarily in that order. Try to concentrate on what you are getting back for your efforts to quit and give yourself a treat or reward.

Increased appetite

Nicotine tends to suppress your appetite. So it is no wonder that the lack of nicotine will make you feel hungry. The cravings themselves may be interpreted as hunger. You may find you're unusually hungry because your body is in a state of repair and needs more energy than usual. Weight gain is common when people quit smoking. This is caused by the combined effects of changes in your metabolism, increased appetite, improved sense of taste and often by replacing cigarettes with snacking. Watching your diet, eating low calorie foods and increasing the level of exercise will help. Fresh fruit, dried fruit and fruit juices are all great sources of natural energy and won't pile on the pounds. Weight management is discussed in more detail in Chapter 9.

Feeling light-headed or dizzy

Light-headedness may occur as the level of carbon monoxide in the blood starts to fall and oxygen supply to the brain increases. Dizziness can result from lowered blood pressure (your heart doesn't have to work as hard as it used to) and an increase in the level of oxygen that is reaching the nerves and tissues. These symptoms pass quickly, usually within a few days, and are a good sign that your body is getting more oxygen.

Sore tongue and mouth ulcers

Probably a result of chemical and bacterial changes in the mouth, see a dentist if they persist for longer than a few weeks.

Tingling sensations in your hands and feet

Many people experience headaches and tingling. This is because blood vessels all over your body are opening up and more blood is getting to your brain. Tingling sensations in your hands and feet are a positive sign that your circulation is improving. Your extremities may start to feel warmer. Many smokers notice the skin on their face looks better and improves in colour.

Tiredness

Around 25 per cent of people who quit say they feel unusually tired. In some cases this could be due to disturbed sleep patterns. However, it may also be because of a lack of nicotine. Nicotine is a stimulant and speeds up your body's metabolism to unnaturally high levels. When you stop using tobacco, your metabolism needs to adjust and this may cause a drop in energy levels. If you are at home, take a nap or go to bed early. If you're at work and feeling sleepy, drink a glass of water and take a quick walk outside to help you stay alert.

All these symptoms are normal and will eventually pass. However, if they persist or you are at all worried and want advice, contact your GP or call the NHS Smoking Helpline.

Craving by association

You can crave nicotine and feel irritable long after it has left your bloodstream. This is because many years of smoking can affect the parts of the brain linked to feelings of pleasure. If you have smoked for 10 years with 20 puffs a day you'll have linked the emotional sight, smells and feelings to the relief you get from easing your craving. Many smokers say that they don't know what to do with their hands when they stop and find it hard to finish a meal before they want to light up.

People deal with these symptoms of withdrawal in different ways. Some choose to keep themselves busy with activities they enjoy. Others find it useful to avoid situations they associate with smoking such as restaurants and pubs.

❯ The road to recovery

Day one
Your blood pressure has returned to normal and carbon monoxide has been eliminated from your body.

Day two
Nicotine is no longer detectable in your body. Your skin is getting warmer and your sense of taste and smell are improving.

Day three
This day may be the worst for withdrawal symptoms but be strong and remind yourself that things can only get better now. Once today is over, your symptoms steadily fade away. In three weeks' time, physical withdrawal should be a thing of the past. Keep busy, keep focused.

Day four
You may be feeling restless and empty. This is your body craving nicotine and it is easy to confuse with physical hunger. Drink as much water as you can and keep healthy snacks to hand. Try going for a quiet walk in the park or going to the gym for a workout.

Day five
By now, your breathing will be easier, your skin and eyes should be clearer and you should already feel your energy levels improving. Try to get into the habit of relaxing, morning and night, using a relaxation technique.

Week one

Your sleeping pattern should return to normal. You may find you have a sore throat and are coughing more than usual as your lungs do their job and reject the tar and debris that has accumulated over the years. This is a good sign.

Week two

Blood vessels all over your body are beginning to open up again and your circulation is starting to improve. It will continue to do so for the next few months and your energy levels will quickly rise.

❯ Top tips

- Your body starts to recover as soon as you stub out your last cigarette.
- Nicotine leaves your body completely within 48 hours.
- Focus on what you are gaining, not what you are 'losing'.
- Give yourself frequent non-food rewards.
- To cope with sudden cravings, breathe in deeply and let the air out gently, then slowly sip a glass of water.
- Drink lots of water and eat plenty of fruit, vegetables and fibre-rich food to avoid constipation.
- Cut down on stimulants such as tea or coffee.
- Go out for a walk and get fresh air and exercise to aid concentration.
- Sprinkle lavender oil on the pillow and try a herbal sleep preparation to aid sleep.
- Eat plenty of fresh fruit and vegetables, dried fruit and drink fruit juices.

Chapter 9
Managing Weight Gain

A lot of people worry that when they stop smoking they'll start putting on weight. Some smokers even put off the decision to quit simply because of this fear. While it's true that you can gain a few pounds after you stop smoking, it's important to keep sight of the bigger picture. A couple of extra pounds may seem like a big deal, but it's nothing compared to the damage you'll do by carrying on smoking. Worries about gaining weight should never be an excuse to stay hooked to an addiction that could kill you.

Studies have shown that initial weight gains tend to peak after six months and many people return to their normal weight within a year of quitting the habit. Even if you do put on weight, the benefits to your health from giving up smoking far outweigh the costs. Everyone can control weight through exercise and diet, so when you give up smoking it may just mean eating different, healthier foods and being more active. This chapter can help you plan ways to manage your weight.

A smoker's story

'At work I have only a short tea break so it makes it easier not to go outside for a cigarette. It has also helped going to a group session. I kept myself busy. I learnt the hard way not to compensate for cigarettes by eating more food, so don't make that mistake.' L. Flegg

Get physical

Ex-smokers who take up regular physical exercise have a greater chance of controlling their weight than those who don't. Exercise doesn't need to be complicated – try taking the stairs instead of the lift, or get off the bus a stop or two earlier and walk the rest of your journey. Remember that once you've stopped smoking you'll find being physically active much easier and this will help you to lose any extra weight! There are more ideas on how to keep active later in this next chapter.

Planning a Healthy Diet

First let's look at how to manage weight gain using basic healthy diet principles. To start I'll look at the changes that giving up smoking has made to your relationship with food, and suggest a few simple diet changes that can help to tackle the problems that arise. There are more healthy-eating suggestions later in this chapter.

Nicotine no longer suppresses your appetite?

Studies have shown that when nicotine reaches the brain it causes chemicals such as adrenaline be to released. This, in turn, increases your heart rate and pushes excess glucose into the bloodstream. Nicotine may also inhibit the release of insulin, which is responsible for removing excess sugar from the blood. The result is that smokers can have higher blood sugar levels than non-smokers. Blood sugar acts as an appetite suppressant which may explain why some smokers don't feel hungry as often as non-smokers. To help keep your blood sugar stable and keep you full, eat more fruits, fibre, vegetables and whole grain foods.

Your body doesn't burn calories so fast

When nicotine reaches the brain it causes chemicals to be released that speed your heart rate and increase your metabolic rate (the rate at which the body caries out chemical processes). This means your food is quickly converted to energy and less likely to be stored as fat. When you stop smoking, your body has to readjust to a lower metabolic rate. As your food is now burnt at a slower rate, it is more likely to be stored as fat. Again, try eating more fruits, vegetables, fibre and whole grains. These foods are low in calories and make you feel full for longer.

Food tastes better now

Years of smoking have dulled your appreciation of food. Once your senses of taste and smell recover, it can be surprising to find just how nice food really tastes. As eating becomes a real pleasure again, there is a temptation to overindulge. To avoid this, keep a close watch on your diet, cut down on foods high in fat and sugar and increase your level of exercise. In the first few weeks, try to make small changes to your diet, such as having fruit instead of high-calorie snacks.

You need to fill the need for oral satisfaction

It's possible that putting food in your mouth could become a substitute for the action of smoking. Eating food can bring an immediate feeling of comfort and well-being and, if you are experiencing nicotine withdrawal, eating can bring relief. The trick is to find a balance and not to let snacking get out of hand. Try eating pieces of fruits, or pieces of raw vegetables with low-fat dips, instead of crisps or chocolates.

A smoker's story

'I was really shocked after 17 years of smoking how much I used cigarettes to help me cope with just about everything. It seemed as if all my emotional comfort was tied into the habit. I'd learnt to react to everything by lighting a cigarette. When I was happy, I'd celebrate by lighting up. When I was angry, smoking calmed me down. When I was tired, smoking helped me stay awake. When I was hungry, smoking took the pang away. I cannot think how many times I skipped food. So I guess it's no surprise that without the appetite suppressant I have put on loads of weight.' Lynne Hughes.

◯ Prepare for a new you

If you want to avoid weight gain, it makes sense to eat properly from the start. Up to 70 per cent of an ex-smoker's weight gain is due to increased calorie intake, often through replacing smoking with high-calorie snacking, so avoiding dramatic changes to eating habits is important. When you stop, how about starting a healthy eating programme at the same time. Steer clear of high-calorie, high-fat foods, such as fried foods, and avoid developing bad snacking habits such as eating chocolate instead of smoking.

If you can face up to the challenges of your diet right from the beginning, you won't set up new habits that could make you put on weight. Try this exercise. Imagine yourself as you'd like to look when you have stopped smoking and when you are choosing food, ask yourself:

'Would I be eating this   if I hadn't just stopped smoking?'

If the answer is 'no' you may want to reconsider your choice and reach for healthier snacks like dried fruits. If you've already started to eat, maybe chew slowly on a small mouthful to satisfy the urge but don't eat it all. Picture yourself as the healthy non-smoker you wish to become. Each time you choose some food ask yourself...

'Will eating this   help me achieve my desired self-image?'

List the times that you eat even though you're not hungry

1	
2	
3	

These answers will help you to identify the times you need to distract yourself, for example by being more active. Find something practical to occupy your hands and mind to take your attention away from eating. Take up mentally challenging puzzles like Suduko, gardening, craft work or DIY home repairs. Try to do something physical every day. As you recover from the effects of smoking you'll find this easier. It will help you burn off the calories and control your appetite. Also look at the suggestion for healthy snacks on page 154.

Practical steps

Always plan meals ahead, that way you avoid last-minute high-fat choices or takeaway meals. Eat three regular healthy meals a day, with plenty of complex carbohydrates such as wholemeal bread, whole grain cereals, pasta to keep your appetite under control and reduce the desire to snack. When eating, try to concentrate on each mouthful and notice each taste, colour, smell and texture of the food. Eat slowly. To beat the craving for an after-meal cigarette, leave the table and do something else as soon as you finish eating.

Keep an eating diary

One of the best ways to stop excess weight gain is to avoid making dramatic changes to your eating habits. To see if your decision to stop smoking has affected your diet pattern, keep a food diary to record all the main meals and snacks you had during the week before you quit and compare this with the week after you gave up.

Food Diary 1 (before I quit)

Use the following food diary to record your eating habits before you stopped smoking.

	Time of day
Monday	
Tuesday	
Wednesday	
Thursday	
Friday	
Saturday	
Sunday	

Food Diary 2 (after I quit)

Use the following food diary to record your eating habits now that you have stopped.

	Time of day
Monday	
Tuesday	
Wednesday	
Thursday	
Friday	
Saturday	
Sunday	

This exercise should help you assess any changes you have made to your diet since you quit. In particular, look to see if you are eating more sweets, crisps, chocolates, biscuits, and high-fat or fried foods than before. Try to be honest with yourself or you risk an unpleasant surprise when you next step on the scales.

Shopping guide

A good tip is not to go shopping when you are hungry. You are more likely then to buy high-calorie/high-fat foods. If you fill your supermarket basket with tempting but unhealthy products you're setting yourself up to put on weight.

Eating out

When eating out, skip the first course. Choose low-fat meals and have extra vegetables. Avoid rich sauces and fried or roasted potatoes. A good tip is to share a dessert with a friend. That way you enjoy the taste of pudding but halve your calorie intake!

Drink water

Water is a great craving buster. It can stop you feeling hungry and helps flush out the toxins from smoking. By keeping yourself well hydrated, you'll feel better in general too.

A smoker's story

'I changed my diet to avoid putting on weight. I started a healthy eating plan, making plenty of fresh soup and fruit salads. Cutting up the fruit and vegetables, replaced my need to smoke. Playing compulsive computer games at crunch times after meals kept me occupied. This, combined with walking, has really helped. If I ever got tempted, I asked myself, "Do you want to be an old lady with a cigarette?" The answer was "No". I am still proud now, three years on, and I can laugh now without coughing!' Norma Cooper

---

More tips for cutting calories

The following are for general guidance and you'll know best how to adapt them into your lifestyle. Some ideas may work better than others, depending on your personal circumstances. Whatever you do, don't be too hard on yourself or apply the rules too rigidly as it may make you want to rebel.

- **Switch from full-fat milk to semi-skimmed.**
- **Use a low-fat spread instead of butter.**
- **Use half-fat cheese and grate the cheese – it goes a lot further.**
- **Grill food instead of frying.**
- **Cut out chocolates and biscuits.**
- **Choose wholemeal brown rice and pasta instead of white, as these foods will satisfy your hunger for longer.**
- **Make some sugar-free ice pops to keep in the fridge.**
- **Have a banana or baked apple with your morning coffee instead of biscuits.**

Try some healthy snacks

When you're feeling peckish it is normal to look for a snack. It's a good idea to stock up on some sensible low-calorie snacks – and keep them within reach. That way, when the desire to eat strikes, you can grab something healthy. It doesn't have to be rabbit food, try some of the following tasty ideas. (Put a ✔ by those you think sound appealing.)

- ○ **Low calorie popcorn.**
- ○ **Carrot sticks.**
- ○ **Sunflower seeds.**
- ○ **Dried fruit, including raisins, apricots, apple, banana.**
- ○ **Sugar-free sweets or jelly.**
- ○ **Frozen berries – grapes, raspberries, blueberries.**
- ○ **Herbal teas.**
- ○ **Fresh fruit.**
- ○ **Breadsticks or rice cakes.**
- ○ **Low-fat rice pudding/ready-made custard.**
- ○ **Baked apple with raisins.**

Join a local slimming group

If you need some extra support, you could join a local slimming group. You'll probably find you are not the only ex-smoker struggling with weight gain after stopping smoking, and you may make some new non-smoking friends.

❯ Frequently asked questions

Should I go on a strict diet and stop smoking at the same time?

Stopping smoking is such an important goal the answer is 'NO!' It is better to concentrate on making one major change in your life at a time. The evidence suggests that it is better to tackle smoking as your first priority and then address the issue of weight gain if you need to. When people stop smoking they sometimes make decisions to sort out other aspects of their life as well. There's nothing wrong with this, but you need to take it slowly. Stopping smoking is a huge accomplishment. If you take on too many self-improvement projects at once you could be setting yourself up for hard work. It may be better to set a future date to do the other things you also want to accomplish.

Should I avoid alcohol?

Alcohol is high in calories and can weaken your resolve to stop smoking for good. If you are a regular drinker, a good tip is to space alcoholic drinks by having a glass of water or a non-alcoholic beverage between them. Try to limit your use of alcohol – or avoid it altogether – during the early days because its likely to trigger your urge to smoke.

An ex-smoker's story

'I had just turned 40 and had experienced a nasty health scare. I was smoking 15 cigarettes a day (sometimes 20 at the weekends). I was also overweight and generally unhealthy. I desperately wanted to quit smoking and had

---

a few failed attempts behind me. I always started smoking again because I put on weight. I knew this time, to be successful, I would have to plan a weight loss regime alongside my attempt to quit smoking. I did not want to fail again. I joined the stop-smoking classes at my local NHS group and read up about healthy eating plans. I then bought a relaxation CD to listen to as I went to sleep and got started. I have not looked back. Each day that I stayed smoke-free gave me such a feeling of success and pride that I simply wanted to carry on. I was also losing weight and my skin became clearer. I had much more energy and life was and is to this day getting better and better.'
Andrea Dean

Keeping Active

Exercise is a great way to beat cravings and helps reduce stress and depression. Regular exercise of 30 minutes at least three days a week is enough to improve your fitness level. Sixty minutes of exercise daily will help you lose weight or maintain your weight. Find something active you enjoy doing and phase it in slowly, especially if you haven't been doing much before. For example, instead of going for one 30-minute walk, try two 15-minute walks. Add variety to your route and as you get used to this level of activity, try to walk more.

Walking will clear your mind and help you feel more positive. You will also notice your lung capacity improving. Why not buy a pedometer? This will help you monitor the amount of additional walking you are doing and see if you need to do more. Aim each week to gradually increase your daily number of steps, and work towards a goal of 10,000 steps a day.

Common benefits of exercise

Exercise is good for weight loss, and has the added benefit of releasing endorphins – the feel-good chemical. Common benefits include:

- Reduced stress.
- Reduced weight.
- More stamina.
- Better health.
- Increased feelings of well-being.
- Increased self-esteem and sense of accomplishment.
- Improved muscle tone and physical appearance.
- Improved sleep.
- Improved performance at work.
- Improved mental attitude and general disposition.

Important daily activities

If you prefer, there are numerous day-to-day activities that will burn-off calories and help keep you fit. Even housework counts! Try walking a neighbour's dog for a change of pace.

- Walking.
- Climbing stairs.
- Gardening.
- Housework/cleaning.
- Lifting.

An ex-smoker's story

'When I did my annual fitness test at work I was really surprised to be told my heart rate was taking much longer to recover after exercise than was normal for someone of my age. The doctor advised me to stop smoking but I didn't want to. I was slim and healthy and couldn't see the point. Then my father was diagnosed with emphysema from smoking and I saw the risk I was taking. I stopped with the help of NRT but found going for a brisk walk worked best to beat the cravings. Soon I was out every day, in all weathers, which was not like me at all! Exercise really took my mind off it. At the next annual check-up my body responded as if it was biologically younger. Stopping smoking had made me fitter and the tests proved it.'
Janet Pratt

Becoming more active

Look at your weekly diary and work out the best time to exercise. For example, it might be first thing in the morning, or lunch hour, or early evening. Your normal schedule may have to change but you should be able to find an extra two to three hours a week for exercise. Remember, if you were a 20-a-day smoker, you now have a couple of hours spare with every day.

Some GPs and other health professionals offer an exercise referral scheme that gives people a prescription to access the facilities at a local fitness centre. If you are eligible to join this NHS scheme, you will be offered a physical assessment and a personalised training programme by the centre staff. A course normally lasts 24 sessions and most people attend twice a week.

Joining a local exercise group might be a great way to make new friends! Your local newspaper will have lists of all the various activities taking place in your area. The reference section of your library is also a great place to get ideas of ways to occupy your spare time. If you prefer to stay in, there are lots of different types of exercise videos and DVDs available for home use. Look on the Internet for suitable titles.

Tips for healthy and enjoyable exercising

- **Try out different kinds of exercise.**
- **Exercise regularly, ideally at least five times each week.**
- **Do at least 30 minutes on exercise days.**
- **Three 10-minute spells of exercise a day are as good as a single 30-minute session.**
- **Don't work too hard – exercise at a level where you feel comfortable and can still hold a slightly breathy conversation.**
- **Your breathing should be a little faster than usual and you will feel warmer.**
- **The old saying 'no pain, no gain' is a myth.**
- **Don't be frightened to speak to the fitness instructors at the gym, they're there to help.**

- Exercise regularly and make it a vital part of your lifestyle.
- A physical activity diary can help you plan ahead and set aside time for being active.
- Invest in correct clothing and shoes. Comfort, safety and practicality are important.

Organisations and clubs

There are many sports and activity organisations that can help you increase your fitness levels and take your mind off smoking. Why not try out martial arts such as t'ai chi, kick-boxing and judo? Or something completely different such as ice skating.

Get dancing

Perhaps you fancy yourself as a dancing champion! If so, why not look for a class specialising in salsa, jazz, jive or tango. If you want more of a group activity, line dancing is popular.

Get about – indoors and out

If you prefer a breath of fresh air then you could always join the National Ramblers Association and take part in a countryside walk. You will find local walks of varying distances classified from leisurely to strenuous.

For a more relaxing exercise option indoors, perhaps you could try out a yoga or Pilates class. Again check your local newspaper or library for a class near you. Swimming is another excellent form of cardiovascular exercise and your local library will have a list of council-run swimming pools in your area.

An ex-smoker's story

'I used to be a club standard athlete competing all year round in both cycling and running events. Unfortunately, I've suffered a bad back for most of my life which eventually led to me getting a prolapsed disc. I had to take an extended rest from exercise. Eventually I had an operation on my back and was mobile enough to start gentle exercise again. My goal was to get fit enough to

complete a long-distance race. My first thought wasn't about giving up smoking but I found the more I exercised the less I wanted to smoke. I decided to set myself a six- month quit smoking plan! With the help of NRT, regular running, cycling and working out in the gym, I'm almost there. I've even completed my first race three months ahead of schedule. My lungs feel a lot healthier, I no longer crave cigarettes and working towards my goal has helped me get my confidence back and beat my depression.' Gary Bruce

Where can you go to get started?

To start a more active life – check out the following ideas:

BBC Health and Fitness

This site www.bbc.co.uk/health/fitness/index.shtml covers all aspects of health and fitness and gives advice on suitable clothing and preparations for your chosen sport.

Cycling

Cycling is another excellent form of exercise. The governing body for British cycling has launched a new initiative called Everyday Cycling, aimed at getting the nation active on bikes by providing fun and exciting cycling opportunities and incentives for people of all ages and abilities. Visit their website for more details on www.everydaycycling.com.

Football Association

Our national sport is available for both men and women and the FA website gives details on activities at a local level. Find out how you can get involved by logging on to: www.thefa.com.

Golf

This sport can be started at any age. It is an excellent form of gentle exercise and requires concentration – the perfect way to take your mind off cigarettes. Most councils run local 9- or 18-

hole courses where you pay by the day and don't have to be a member. Golf lessons are a great way to begin. Check out your local driving range or course and ask for details.

Green Gym

This is a unique health group that exercises its participants in the countryside or open spaces. With the Green Gym you can become fitter and healthier by taking part in conservation activities such as:

○ **Tree Planting.**

○ **Creating school nature areas.**

○ **Hedge laying.**

○ **Constructing dry stone walls, fences, gateways and stiles.**

It offers a new way to get fit and healthy, providing an exciting alternative for people who do not like the idea of joining a sports centre or gym. As well as improving your health, by taking part you will have the opportunity to meet new people and learn new skills. There is also the satisfaction of knowing that you are making a difference to your environment. For more details contact their website on: www.greengym.org.uk.

Judo

Judo training is an ideal form of exercise as it serves as a great cardiovascular workout, improves stamina as well as general health and overall fitness. Physical strength and flexibility will also be improved as a direct result of trying to control and dictate the movement of your opponent. Your balance and posture will also be enhanced as well as improved mental reaction time. The British Judo Association's website www. britishjudo.org.uk will give you details of a class local to you.

Line dancing

Line dancing is a very social form of exercise, where you can meet people and make new friends while exercising. Another advantage of line dancing is that you don't need a partner and so won't feel out of place if you go alone. The leader provides the advice and tuition and some lively country and western music. No special equipment is needed but many regulars wear jeans and boots. It's great fun and suitable for people of all ages and abilities. For details, visit: www.linedancing.org.uk.

National Ramblers Association

There are over five hundred Ramblers Groups which promote walking and improve conditions for walkers at a local level. The association also organises hundreds of group walks a week. These groups are organised into areas and include special walks run and operated at a local level. To find out more about the association or locate your nearest group, visit the website on: www.ramblers.org.uk.

Walking for Health (WHI)

The WHI website www.whi.org.uk is for everyone with an interest in 'walking for health'. It offers information, support and encouragement to complete beginners, existing walkers and health and leisure professionals.

Yoga

The British Wheel of Yoga is the largest yoga organisation in the country and has been running for 40 years. There is a nation-wide network of over 3,000 qualified teachers and the website promotes yoga classes to the general public. For information, visit the website on: www.bwy.org.uk.

Go for it!

Incorporating all or even some of the above as part of your everyday life can dramatically increase your levels of fitness and burn off excess calories. Work out what is best for you. You can exercise in all kinds of different ways and finding something you really enjoy will help you to continue.

I plan to increase my general activity levels by

- ☐
- ☐
- ☐

I have decided to try the following new ways exercise

- ☐
- ☐
- ☐

Top tips

- Remember, gaining a little weight is a minor health risk compared to smoking.
- Take regular exercise and keep active.
- Avoid chocolate bars and high-fat food.
- Try sugar-free chewing gum, air-popped popcorn or dried berries.
- Keep occupied with puzzles, gardening, craft work or DIY.
- Eat regular meals with plenty of complex carbohydrates to control your appetite and reduce the urge to snack.
- Drink more water to ease your cravings and make you feel better.
- Make plenty of healthy low-calorie snacks and keep them within reach.
- Call the NHS Smoking Helpline for more tips and support on 0800 169 0 169.
- Exercise with a friend or join a local gym.
- Choose a form of physical activity or exercise you really enjoy.
- When you get the chance, use the stairs and walk or cycle in favour of lifts, escalators and cars.

Chapter 10
Staying Stopped –
For Good!

Congratulations! You've managed the first two weeks of your quit smoking plan. You really need and deserve to give yourself a treat for this effort. Don't underestimate this achievement. Some people fail after just three days, but you are going strong, so celebrate. How about using some of the money you've saved to spoil yourself?

The next few weeks are going to be an interesting time because you are learning to adapt to a lifestyle that does not include tobacco. It's not an understatement to say you are learning a new way to live your life. By now you will have noticed that there are some situations you need to prepare for to avoid temptation. For example, have you been offered a cigarette and almost taken one before remembering you've quit?

You have made a tremendous effort to have got this far and there is absolutely no reason why you cannot go even further. You can stay smoke free and achieve your goal. There is no magic date after stopping when you'll know for sure you're never going to smoke again. Some people feel like this after a couple of weeks while others spend years 'resisting'. This chapter will prepare you to turn your back on smoking forever.

An ex-smoker's story

'I thought I'd been careful and that my two children didn't know I smoked. I'd be rushing round getting them off to bed so I could sneak outside for my ciggy. Finally I decided to stop. Two weeks after I quit, I was surprised when my daughter said, "Mummy, what's happened? Are

you OK? You've been so nice to us for the last few weeks."
I had to stop and think what she meant. Then I realised
that when all I thought about was getting my smoke break
I must have been really cranky with them at bedtime. She
meant that because the pressure was off to go and smoke,
I'd been reading bedtime stories and playing games with
them. This is a benefit of stopping smoking that I hadn't
expected.' Yvonne Peters

❯ You're in the driving seat

When you started on this journey you had some very strong
reasons for giving up cigarettes and expected some benefits
for your effort. By now you'll know it's possible to live without
cigarettes. Your old habits are gradually being replaced by new
ones and you are learning to resist temptation. You've certainly
turned the first corner and the good news is that the trip will
start to get easier. As signs of withdrawal leave your body you'll
become healthier, more energetic and your skin will look better.
Be reassured you can live a happy, full and rewarding life as a
non-smoker. You are not losing anything; you are saving your life
and your money. Cigarettes never were your friend. Every one of
the people I've nursed who were ill from smoking regretted what
they had done to themselves.

If you started smoking when you were young, it's likely you've
never experienced a day of your adult life without smoking. No
wonder it takes effort to separate yourself from the habit. Just
remember you are saying goodbye to a habit that could kill you.
You've started to replace smoking and live a different life. You're
regaining control.

An ex-smoker's story

'I had smoked for 20 years – only stopping while I was pregnant. I then stopped smoking when I had a really bad chest infection. Having rarely been off sick, I was off work for three weeks. I was sitting out on my children's swing, trying to smoke outside so the family wouldn't know. I found it hard to breathe and realised just how ridiculous the whole situation was. I decided there and then to give up. I used the patches and I stayed on them for three months, steadily reducing the doses. I've now been an ex-smoker for four years. I used to get a chest infection every winter and spring, now I rarely get ill, a simple cold at most. I've noticed lots of benefits. My singing voice in the choir is much clearer. I sing high soprano and can now reach the notes easily – even breath holds are no problem for the longer phrases. I'm still thankful I stopped. This is reinforced on a daily basis when I see colleagues at work racing to get to the smoking room to have a quick puff. That used to be me.' Karen Love

You have chosen to go smoke free and there are many others who have been on the journey ahead of you. In the UK today, there are more people who have given up smoking than there are smokers. No one is saying it's easy, but having done it you can reap the rewards. You may even become an example to your friends and family who want to stop smoking. Other smokers know how hard it is to quit and will be proud of you. They'll ask, 'How did you do it? What worked for you?'

An ex-smoker's story

'If someone would have said to me four months ago that I would now be a non-smoker who has also lost two stone in weight and is enjoying every minute of her life, I would have assumed one of two things – either I'd lost my hearing or they'd lost their mind!' Andrea Dean

You made a great decision when you decided to stop. The only decision you have to make now is to stay stopped. To help you avoid sabotaging your goal, even unconsciously, try doing the interactive exercises on the following pages.

Reinforcing your new habits

Due to past conditioning, you may still respond to a current situation with an old instinct. This may give you an urge to have a cigarette. But you've chosen to change this 'gut' reaction. Remember that if you gave in and smoked, the 'urge' would simply come back within a few hours. Only this time there wouldn't need to be an external stimulus. Your body, having received the nicotine buzz once again, will simply want it again...and again! Having a cigarette will not take away the issue or problem. It will just add to the list of things you need to deal with at a later stage. It is the urge to smoke that you need to address, not the lack of cigarettes in your life.

A smoke-free life

Stopping smoking is a long-term investment, so be patient with yourself. Continue to take it one day at a time and you'll soon be proud of your achievement. Ex-smokers often talk about what they 'gave up' – so change that thought right now. You are NOT giving up anything that was worth having and you are gaining a lot. By not smoking, you are giving your body the best present it could ever have. It helps to remember that we ascribe too much power to cigarettes. They can't change anything or make things better. As Freud said, 'Sometimes, a cigarette is just a cigarette.'

An ex-smoker's story

'My tip for quitters is...remember when you had your first drag? It was bloody awful wasn't it? But you battled on to look good and become a smoker...well, put as much effort into stopping the habit as you did to start. I believe that before anybody even tries to quit they must identify an

incentive, a driving force, something they can call upon when things are tough and it will still be powerful enough to work for them. My ambition is to grow into a fit and healthy old lady who still enjoys walking in the country and can keep up with the best of them. I'm 25 now and want to look so good that people will be in disbelief at my age! Since quitting, I don't feel the cold as much. I don't get those white, dead cold fingers any more and my skin looks better. Set a date. Don't worry about weight gain – you can sort that out later. Put money away that would have gone up in smoke. Use the aids and support that is available from your local smoking cessation service. Tell people you're a non-smoker – it sounds good!' Mai Rees

Focus on the gains

To stop and stay stopped you need to keep a strong and focused mind. Reminding yourself that you are in control, combined with a positive mental attitude, will help you stay stopped – and enjoy life as a non-smoker! Focus on the benefits you are already experiencing:

Physical benefits

O You breathe more easily.

O Your risk of serious disease is starting to fall.

O Your blood vessels are beginning to reopen and your circulation improving.

O Your energy levels are rising as carbon monoxide leaves your body.

O Your skin is warming up and beginning to glow again.

O You have a better chance of conceiving and of having a healthy pregnancy and baby.

O You have no more stinging, watery eyes due to your own tobacco smoke.

Lifestyle benefits

- You live in a cleaner, fresher house.
- You can say goodbye to cigarette holes in your clothes and cigarette burns on your furniture.
- You no longer put those around you at risk.
- You have healthier children who are less likely to start smoking.
- You are spending less.
- You'll become a lot richer!

Social benefits

- Your food tastes better.
- You are more attractive to potential partners.
- Your clothes, hair, breath and skin no longer smell.
- You can go out and enjoy yourself without having to smoke.

Emotional benefits

- You have more confidence and self-esteem, knowing you've had the determination and willpower to give up.
- You feel more alive and positive.

Now think about how good you're going to feel in a few months' time. You'll be living a smoke-free life, you'll feel healthier and have more control over your time.

> An ex-smoker's story
>
> *'When I was smoking I started to lose my sense of smell – I couldn't smell a bunch of flowers or even my food. My breathing was becoming difficult too. I wanted to give up smoking to enjoy my health, enjoy my own family and watch my grandchildren growing up. I found gardening really helped to take my mind off cigarettes. I've even started going to the gym and now feel much healthier, which motivates me and helps me avoid the temptation to smoke.'* Vincenzo Iacolino

⟩ Guard against temptation

When you first quit smoking, the decision will have been on your mind most of the time. This is normal. The greatest risk comes as your new daily routines are being consolidated, so put some safeguards in place to protect against relapse. Whenever you make new social arrangements, check you're not walking into a temptation zone. This is still a sensitive time and you're learning to integrate a new lifestyle. Be careful about which invitations you accept and whose company you keep.

Most smokers will tell you that it's the things they didn't plan for that caught them out. It's really important to work out these details beforehand. Memories and associations may tempt you. Be kind to yourself. Most habits take years to form, so it's natural to feel out of sorts in some places while learning to become smoke free.

An ex-smoker's story

'My main temptation was nights out in the pub with friends who smoke. It wasn't easy at first if they lit up but I found that if I went to talk to someone who wasn't smoking, I could cope. I appreciate the fact that I don't smell of smoke any more and have got used to having more money. I've found it was important to do something better to occupy my time when I gave up smoking. I joined a gym, which has also helped me control my weight.' Jo Colls

---

Do a 'temptation assessment'

List the places you are concerned about visiting without smoking.

You've started the journey but it's very easy to double back – so keep that list of reasons of why you are stopping close at hand. Look for ways you can get more support. Maybe the novelty of giving up smoking has worn off for your family and friends, but you've still got to carry on day by day. Speak to people you know who have already stopped smoking and talk about how you're feeling. If in any doubt, get reassurance. Ask them how they're feeling now they've successfully quit the habit.

An ex-smoker's story

'I started to smoke at around 15. When Mum discovered my habit she popped a note in my pack of ten saying "1 leads to 2, 2 leads to 3, 3 leads to 5 and 5 leads you to a habit of a lifetime that smells awful, costs a fortune and will make you ill." I carried on because I knew best, after all I was 15! I've often wanted to stop, but problems in my life such as separations, divorce, family bereavements, stress and work always kept me clutching to the packet. Last year I heard these words from the apple of my eye: "Dad, I don't want you to die of cancer. What would I do without you?" This finally kick-started me into taking "giving up" seriously. I'm now cross that I've waited until I'm 39 with a smelly habit, no money and a bad cough to realise Mum was right. I took my last drag as the clocks struck 12 on New Year's Eve and have not looked back.'
Graham Dukes

Avoid false memory syndrome

After you've quit, your memories are likely to be mixed, both of sadness and joy. Some people think of their past life as a smoker with disgust and others wish they could invent a safe cigarette so they could go back to the habit. Don't be a hostage to memories. Some things are better left in the past, and dirty ashtrays, stale smoke and tar-stained walls are some of them. If you forget the reality, there is a danger you'll focus on your rosy memories and start wishing you could be back there.

Take a reality check

Stopping smoking can be like ending a love affair, the time wasn't right, ultimately the person wasn't right, but that doesn't stop you wishing you could have it all back again to give it another go. In these situations people may invent different endings and play an 'I wish' game. If you do this with smoking you'll create a desire to smoke. If you're bored or at a crunch point, you may dwell on 'false' memories of your 'love' of smoking. Instead, frame your thoughts on smoking in a realistic way.

Memories are made of...fag ash

Visualise a full ashtray you've had to empty. A smoke-filled room after a party that needs to be cleaned and aired. Remember the smell and how the room looked. Think of times you've been ill and coughing. Or when you've suddenly needed to exert yourself and found that your body doesn't respond quickly. These are the memories to hold onto instead of the delights of smoking. They're the truth.

very seriously. You need to be strong – really strong – to ignore the temptations at particular times, such as early morning, after meals and so on. I also found it important not to run away from my smoking friends, staying with them actually strengthened my willpower.' Allie Munu

❯ Don't get tripped up by complacency

Many smokers report a danger time at about five or six weeks. Withdrawal symptoms are behind you, you're feeling physically better, mentally more alert and you may have forgotten just how bad you felt when you were still smoking. Some even indulge in fantasies of being able to smoke again – as and when they want. Beware! Complacency is dangerous. Remind yourself that there is no such thing as one cigarette. There never was before and there won't be this time either. Focusing on a specific reward can help to keep up your motivation. Here are some of the reasons people gave for starting smoking again:

- ○ **'I wondered what a cigarette would taste like now.'**
- ○ **'I thought I could get away with having "just one".'**
- ○ **'I said to myself I'm back in control so a few puffs won't matter.'**
- ○ **'I didn't use any treatment to help my withdrawal symptoms and couldn't cope.'**
- ○ **'I hadn't thought about "smoking triggers" and automatically lit up.'**
- ○ **'I didn't plan alternative coping strategies.'**
- ○ **'I hit a bad patch and cigarettes seemed the only answer.'**
- ○ **'I had a personal tragedy.'**
- ○ **'I was putting on too much weight.'**
- ○ **'I became so moody the people around me "made me smoke".'**
- ○ **'I didn't feel "better".'**
- ○ **'My smoking friends and family taunted me.'**
- ○ **'I decided it wasn't worth the effort and just gambled on staying healthy.'**

Replacement thoughts

Dangerous thoughts can sabotage your progress and take you back to where you started. It helps to make plans to counter these thoughts. You may find it useful to work out replacement thoughts such as:

O **'There is no such thing as just one cigarette.'**
O **'I want to stay healthy.'**
O **'I'm free and my time is my own.'**

Now think up your own personal statements to help you counter any temptation to light up.

I will counter any dangerous thoughts by reminding myself

An ex-smoker's story

'I lost both my parents through smoking. Losing both parents is bad enough but to something you can avoid is much worse. It was horrible seeing my parents suffer from cancer. I finally managed to stop because I didn't want my partner and child to see me suffer in the same way.'

Robert Bouse

❯ Prevention strategies

Most smokers are well aware of their tobacco 'hot spots' and temptations. Sometimes, people look for an excuse to start if staying stopped is becoming a problem. Smokers are famous for 'setting up' a situation to give themselves a 'good' reason or excuse to light up. This type of self-sabotage needs to be avoided. This exercise will help you assess your chances of relapse. Answer these following questions:

What would I gain from starting smoking again?

If I'm honest – the things I need to be concerned about are:

I plan to manage these concerns by:

I can ask the following people to help me by:

My strategy to avoid getting caught out is:

What do I need to say to myself if I considered smoking again?

An ex-smoker's story

'First I stopped all smoking in the bedroom and gradually used the same rule in each room of the house. Then I stopped smoking at work. This was great because I never really had time for a whole cig and most of it was going to waste anyway. My colleagues were enjoying the fact that I wasn't running off every hour and in turn they became very supportive of me. If you have a friend or a partner who would like to quit as well, then give up together. It makes a big difference having the support of someone who's going through the same withdrawal symptoms. I spent the money I saved on cigs on beauty treatments. After three weeks of treating myself I never looked back!'
Karina White

⟩ You've done the right thing!

If you ever find yourself contemplating how nice a cigarette would be, or wishing you could light up when you are sitting with a drink, move your thoughts into the present time and create a new picture of yourself, enjoying the drink just as you are – a non-smoker.

Think over your life as it is right now. Remind yourself nothing is missing. Reflecting on the past may trick you into lighting up in order to recreate past feelings. The truth is that, never mind how hard you try, this is impossible. While you still give yourself hope, part of you is holding onto the belief that you can go back to smoking. If necessary remind yourself why you've said goodbye to the habit. Otherwise you're putting yourself in a very tricky predicament. It's like spending all evening looking at the phone, wondering whether to ring them or, even worse, hoping they'll call you.

Changing your mind about the past benefits helps you stay stopped for good. Focus on the present and reject all possibility of having just one.

Say 'hello' to your future

These first few weeks will have given you a greater understanding of the challenge you've taken on and your ability to succeed. You've done so well and hopefully will have lots more confidence in your ability to manage the future. You'll have a smoke-free lifestyle and gained the benefits you want.

How I have rewarded myself for stopping smoking

1	
2	
3	
4	
5	

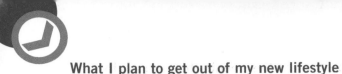

What I plan to get out of my new lifestyle

1	
2	
3	
4	
5	

Taking care of yourself

The following exercise is to encourage you to look at the wider aspects of your life and help you find ways to take even better care of yourself. You may have pushed yourself hard as you went through the process of stopping and might even be feeling that your body is out of balance. So now is a good time to invest in yourself. This is a really important step. If you deposit money in a bank your bank balance will look healthier, which in turn will enhance your credit rating. Investing in yourself will have the effect of enhancing your life. You've started this process by becoming smoke free. Having taken this amazing step, why not ask yourself what you can do next to increase your quality of life.

You've probably already noticed that when you feel happy your thoughts and feelings reflect this and you become much more positive in your outlook. Feeling upbeat definitely opens the doorway to positive events. The better you feel about yourself the less likely you are to be tempted to relapse.

Something nice I plan to do for myself in the future is:

Make a list of all the positive events that happen to you this week

Notice the good things that take place on a day-to-day basis. Include the things that bring a smile to your face or make you feel peaceful, content or excited.

Monday

Tuesday

Wednesday

Thursday

Friday

Saturday

Sunday

Review this list if you have a 'bad' day and want to blame it on your decision to stop smoking. A smoke-free life is more rewarding and healthier and safer.

> **An ex-smoker's story**
>
> *'When I gave up I made a point of saving all the money I would have spent on cigarettes. I kept this going for a year because I had something very special in mind. It was this that stopped me from relapsing. I'd always wanted a car of my own but couldn't afford a large bank loan. Saving up my cigarette money enabled me to buy my own car with a small 'affordable' loan. I've never felt so proud as the day I drove off the forecourt and continued my smoke-free life.'* Roswyn Brown

Achieving lasting success

As time passes, it's possible to forget the effort you put into stopping the habit. Breaking an addiction is no mean feat. You really deserve lots of support and congratulations. Remember, you've learnt to become smoke free.

If you can do this, doesn't it make you wonder what else you can achieve? The following exercise is designed to help you take stock of where you are now and build on your learning and success.

My effort to stop smoking was worthwhile because...

Since I stopped smoking my life has improved because...

I can now look forward to...?

What successfully stopping smoking says about me...

What qualities and strengths helped me stop smoking?

If I can stop smoking, I should also be able to...

An ex-smoker's story

'I'd tried to stop several times before, all without success. I started smoking when I was 18, and now I'm 35. It was a very powerful thought when I realised that soon I would have been a smoker longer then I had been a non-smoker. I no longer wanted to be classed a smoker by my family, friends and colleagues. I told myself that smoking was a stupid thing to continue and stopping would be a life-changing decision. I decided to use both NRT and group support sessions. I think my positive outlook has helped and I have given some inspiration to others that it can be done. My wife, who smoked since the age of 13, stopped last week. I found I gained some weight, and was eating and drinking slightly more than before, but this is manageable, whereas suffering from a smoking-related disease is not. The rapid increase in lung function, sense of smell, and feeling of moral superiority are my powerful incentives to keep going. I've saved £420 in the last three months. I work hard for this money and prefer it to be in my pocket than a cigarette company's.' Graham McLaurin

Top tips

- Reinforce your new non-smoking habits until they become second nature.
- Think how good you feel now and how much better you'll feel in the future.
- Focus on all that you have gained – not on what you have given up.
- List all the good things in your life now that you are a non-smoker.
- Don't get complacent – avoid 'high-risk' situations and continue to use coping strategies.
- Don't give in to temptation – not even one.
- Avoid false memories – your smoking past was never good and your non-smoking future will be much, much better.
- Replace that old mental image of yourself as a stressed, cigarette-obsessed smoker with a new one as a happy and contented non-smoker.

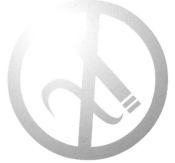

Appendix

⊙ Useful Organisations And Websites

Stop-Smoking Support and Tobacco Information Websites

The following organisations have websites that provide more information on the politics of tobacco, the health consequences of smoking and how to stop.

Action on Smoking and Health (ASH)

www.ash.org.uk

ASH is a campaigning public health charity providing information, reports and publications for professionals and the public. It works to secure public, media, parliamentary, local and national Government support for a comprehensive programme to tackle the epidemic of tobacco-related disease. ASH has successfully campaigned for a ban on tobacco advertising, the provision of stop smoking services, and for smoking to be banned in workplaces and public places. ASH campaigns for effective public health policies, including initiatives to help people quit. It also highlights the activities of the tobacco industry and presses for enforcement of current legislation. Email: enquiries@ash.org.uk. Telephone:
England: 020 7739 5902
Scotland: 0131 225 4725
Wales: 02 9 2064 1101
Northern Ireland: 02 8 9049 2007

Encams

www.encams.org

This organisation runs the Keep Britain Tidy campaign and offers advice on dealing with cigarette litter.

NHS Stop Smoking Services

www.givingupsmoking. co.uk

This is an online resource with advice, information and support to help you stop smoking and stay stopped.
Helpline: 0800 169 0 169

Local NHS Stop Smoking Services

www.givingupsmoking. co.uk/nhs_sss/find/

This website will help you find your local NHS Stop Smoking Service. You can search by postcode.

Nicotine Anonymous
www.nicotine-anonymous.org

Nicotine Anonymous is a non-profit fellowship of men and women helping each other live nicotine-free lives. The fellowship offers group support and recovery using a 12-step programme adapted from Alcoholics Anonymous. Nicotine Anonymous welcomes all those seeking freedom from nicotine addiction, including those using cessation programmes and nicotine withdrawal aids.

No Smoking Day (NSD)
www.nosmokingday.org.uk

This is the official website for No Smoking Day and the charity that runs it. No Smoking Day itself is held on the second Wednesday in March each year. It aims to help people who want to stop smoking by creating a supportive environment for them and by highlighting the many sources of help available. The NSD website is packed with information to help and encourage smokers to quit.

QUIT
www.quit.org.uk

QUIT is the independent UK charity whose aim is to save lives by helping smokers to stop. The site offers a freephone number for smokers wanting to quit.
Quitline 0800 002200 (9 a.m. – 9 p.m. 7 days a week)

Email counselling stopsmoking@quit.org.uk
Information info@quit.org.uk

QUIT Helpline – Ethnic Languages

QUIT counsellors include speakers of Bengali, Gujarati, Hindi, Punjabi and Urdu offering confidential, friendly help and advice in these languages. Free informative leaflets are also available in all these languages.

Bengali: 0800 002244
(Monday 1–9 p.m.)
Gujarati: 0800 002255
(Tuesday 1–9 p.m.)
Hindi: 0800 002255
(Wednesday 1–9 p.m.)
Punjabi: 0800 002277
(Thursday 1–9 p.m.)
Urdu: 0800 002288
(Sunday 1–9 p.m.)

QUIT for Health Professionals
www.quit.org.uk

QUIT runs training courses for health care professionals on a wide range of smoking issues, including 'smoking and young people', 'smoking and depression' and 'relapse prevention'. The department also runs information sessions within organisations – advising companies on implementing no smoking policies and talking to staff wanting to quit. Visit the website for more details.

Qult Smoking UK
www.quitsmokinguk.com
UK online community for quitting smokers by quitting smokers.

Tobacco FactFile
www.tobaccofactfile.org
Tobacco FactFile presents key facts and data about tobacco.

Treat Tobacco
www.treattobacco.net
This website offers information, help and advice on various tobacco-related topics including finance, health, shopping, dating and business, as well as links to websites.

❯ Charity, General Health and Medical Research Websites

Asthma UK
www.asthma.org.uk
Asthma UK is a charity dedicated to improving the health and well-being of the 5.2 million people affected by asthma in the UK. The charity works with asthma sufferers, health professionals and researchers to develop and share expertise in order to increase understanding of this debilitating condition and reduce its effect on people's lives.

British Dental Association (BDA)
www.bda-dentistry.org.uk
Latest news on dentistry, information for dentists and students and public information.

British Heart Foundation
www.bhf.org.uk
The BHF website promotes healthy living and gives advice on heart health. It explains the risks of smoking and how smoking is not conducive to a healthy heart. The BHF is the UK's leading heart charity and produces a range of literature, posters, leaflets and other resources designed to help smokers to quit. For more than 40 years, the BHF has been at the forefront of the fight against heart disease, funding research, education and care. The foundation also provides life-saving cardiac equipment and support for rehabilitation and patient care.

British Lung Foundation
www.blf-uk.org
The British Lung Foundation is the only charity in the UK dedicated to improving the prevention, diagnosis, treatment and cure of all lung diseases. It produces a range of fact sheets and information, including living with lung cancer, children's lung disease. The British Lung Foundation produces a booklet about stopping smoking, which aims to support smokers through this difficult challenge.

British Medical Association (BMA)
www.bma.org.uk
The BMA is a professional association of doctors, representing their interests and providing services for its 123,000 plus members.

Cancer Research UK
www.cancerresearchuk.org
Cancer Research UK is the largest volunteer-supported cancer research organisation in the world. This site gives user-friendly and up-to-date information on cancer and individual cancers. It includes details of how to get involved with a wide range of events, fundraise, or volunteer. You can also donate online.

Department of Health (DoH)
www.doh.gov.uk
The official Department of Health website, giving the department's policy on smoking, the ban on advertising of tobacco products plus general information on smoking and smoking-related diseases.

Directgov
www.direct.gov.uk
This website provides the latest and widest range of public service information. This is a good starting point for answering your health concerns plus links to health services, information and support groups.

Doctor Patient Partnership (DPP)
www.dpp.org.uk
The DPP is a UK charity and membership organisation.
It aims to encourage better communication between patients and healthcare professionals, promote the responsible use of NHS services and offer practical advice on self-medication.

Foundation for the Study of Infant Deaths (FSID)
www.sids.org.uk/fsid
FSID is one of the UK's leading baby charities working to prevent sudden infant deaths and promote baby health. FSID supports bereaved families, promotes lifesaving information to health professionals and the public and funds research.
Helpline: 0870 787 0554

LifeBytes
www.lifebytes.gov.uk
This website gives young people aged 11–14 facts about health in a fun and interesting way.

Mind, Body & Soul
www.mindbodysoul.gov.uk
This website too gives the lowdown on health for young people, and is aimed at those aged 14–16.

Muslim Health Network (MHN)

www.muslimhealthnetwork.org

The MHN provides information and education on health issues affecting the UK's 1.6 million Muslims. A section called 'Smoke Free Ramadan' provides information on giving up during the holy month of fasting.

National Heart Forum (NHF)

www.nationalheartforum.org.uk

This website includes information about smoking and smoking-related issues such as smoke-free public places, tobacco control and cancer. The job of the NHF is to co-ordinate the around 50 organisations representing professional, consumer, charity and public services involved in coronary heart disease prevention and treatment throughout the UK. Since its launch, the NHF has been instrumental in driving the national coronary heart disease prevention policy agenda, developing consensus and evidence-based recommendations for action across a diverse range of issues and settings and co-coordinating advocacy for their implementation.

NHS Direct

www.nhsdirect.nhs.uk

NHS Direct provides healthcare advice and information for the public.

National Institute for Health and Clinical Excellence (NICE)

www.nice.org.uk

NICE is an independent organisation responsible for providing national guidance on promoting good health and preventing and treating ill health. You can read the guidance on 'The use of Nicotine Replacement Therapy and Bupropion (Zyban) for Smoking Cessation (2002)' on this site.

Royal College of Nursing (RCN)

www.rcn.org.uk

The RCN is the largest nursing organisation in the world. It works in partnership with patients to improve standards of patient care. The RCN Tobacco Education project has been set up to enable nurses to help people stop smoking and also offers advice to nurses who want to quit.

Royal College of Physicians (RCP)
www.rcplondon.ac.uk
The Royal College of Physicians conducts examinations, training, education and research in medicine and advises the Government, public and the profession on health and medical matters. The RCP has a Tobacco Advisory Group and publishes books on the health consequences of tobacco use.

Roy Castle Lung Cancer Foundation
www.roycastle.org
The Roy Castle Lung Cancer Foundation is a UK charity, dedicated to defeating lung cancer. Its work includes research into lung cancer, providing support for those affected by lung cancer and also educates children on this issue. Its community stop smoking service is called Roy Castle Fag Ends. It was started twelve years ago by a group of ex-smokers and has developed to become one of the most successful stop smoking services in England. The service aims to make support to stop smoking universally and immediately accessible. The service runs 'drop in' groups at 43 different venues across Liverpool. These groups are all ongoing, with new people joining each week. Referrals are taken from GPs, health care professionals, the telephone helpline and self-referral.

The Stroke Association
www.stroke.org.uk
The Stroke Association funds research into the causes, prevention, diagnosis and treatment of stroke and into rehabilitation after stroke. The association aims to prevent strokes by informing the public how to reduce the risk of stroke. The association's fact sheet explains how smoking increases the risk of stroke and describes the help and support available if you want to give up smoking.

The Time is Right
www.thetimeisright.co.uk
This sponsored site offers advice, support and information on the difficulties of quitting smoking.

Wired for Health
www.wiredforhealth.gov.uk
Wired for Health, has been developed for teachers in schools to provide information on health and national health policies and initiatives, including the Healthy Schools Programme.

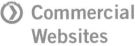

Commercial Websites

GASP Smoke Free Solutions

www.gasp.org.uk

GASP supplies tobacco control resources and consultancy, in the UK and worldwide. It offers over 400 stop-smoking and tobacco-control resources including leaflets, books, educational packs, training manuals, displays, posters, 3D models, carbon monoxide monitors, testing equipment and promotional items for professionals and the public on all aspects of smoking prevention. Catalogues are available by via the website, or email: gasp@gasp.org.uk.

Life Planner by Jennifer Percival

www.thought-catcher.com

After you have succeeded stopping smoking you may feel ready to tackle other issues / areas in your life. Life Planner is a step-by-step guide to helping you find creative solutions and the interactive exercises make it easy for you to plan your next step.

Nicorette

www.nicorette.co.uk

This site is sponsored by the pharmaceutical company Pfizer. As well as giving details on the Nicorette range of nicotine replacement products, this site offers reasons to give up, helpful daily tips and information relating to weight control. It is also possible to download 'desktop diversions' which are games aimed at diverting your attention when you feel the urge to smoke.

Nicotinell

www.nicotinell.com

This site, sponsored by Novartis, includes information about Nicotinell's nicotine replacement therapy in the form of gum, lozenges and patches. Help and advice to quit is offered.

NiQuitin CQ

www.click2quit.co.uk

This site is supported by Glaxosmithkline and offers a 10-week support programme providing tailored stop-smoking advice based on the needs of the individual. The site includes advice, discussion board, testimonials from people that have managed to quit and a 'bad day button' – offering tips to help guide individuals through sticky situations and difficult days.

International Organisations

America

American Lung Association

www.lungusa.org

The American Lung Association is the oldest voluntary health organisation in the United States. Its aim is to fight lung disease in all its forms, with special emphasis on asthma, tobacco control and environmental health.

Florida Truth Campaign

www.wholetruth.com

This website has information about US tobacco manufacturers.

Quit Net US

www.quitnet.org

American community and support site for people trying to give up smoking.

Quit Smoking

www.quitsmoking.about.com

This site is a New York based website to help those wanting to give up smoking. It includes a photo gallery of images showing what smoking does to the body.

Australia

ACOSH (Australian Council on Smoking and Health)

www.acosh.org

ACOSH is a non-government, non-profit organisation which aims to raise awareness on issues relating to smoking and health and lobby tobacco industries and governments in the fight against tobacco.

Action on Smoking and Health Australia

www.ashaust.org.au

The website offers information for smokers and parents of smokers and provides many links to smoking facts and anti-tobacco media coverage.

QuitNow Australia

www.quitnow.info.au

An Australian anti-smoking site – with gory images. Not for the faint hearted.

Quit Victoria

www.quit.org.au

The website offers a step-by-step guide to giving up smoking, interactive quit tools as well as information on quit courses. The Quitline offers advice for those wanting to quit. You can also order a free Quit Pack.
Quitline: 13 7848

OxyGen
www.oxygen.org.au
OxyGen is a website dedicated to informing young people about tobacco and its use in Australia. The website aims to encourage young people to explore all the facts about smoking and the tobacco industry.

Canada
Action on Smoking and Health
www.ash.ca
ASH is Western Canada's leading tobacco control agency and aims to shape local, provincial and national strategies to reduce tobacco use.

Canadian Lung Association
www.lung.ca
A non-profit and volunteer-based health charity, The Lung Association depends on donations from the public to support lung health research, education, prevention and advocacy.

Health Canada
www.hc-sc.gc.ca
Federal Department helping Canadians maintain and improve their health.

Smokingsucks.ca
www.smokingsucks.ca
Website offering tobacco industry and smoking facts, as well as tips and advice on quitting.

Europe
European Network for Smoking Prevention (ENSP)
www.ensp.org
ENSP is an international non-profit association that aims to develop a strategy for co-ordinated action among organisations active in tobacco control in Europe.

European Network of Young People Against Tobacco
www.ktl.fi/portal/english
ENYPAT contributes to the reduction of tobacco use among young people through European-wide collaboration, information exchange and programme building.

South Africa
The Heart and Stroke Foundation South Africa
www.heartfoundation.co.za
A non-pofit company charged with reducing the incidence of cardiovascular disease through education and supporting research.

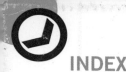

INDEX